YOUR WEIGHT LOSS G-SPOT

*The Woman's How-To Weight Loss System
for a Healthy, Sassy You!*

MICHELLE A. STRONG B.A. (HON), RHN

REGISTERED HOLISTIC NUTRITIONIST

AND

NANCY MILTON CPCC, ACC, PCC

CERTIFIED COACH AND INTENTIONAL COMMUNICATION SPEAKER

Library and Archives Canada Cataloguing in Publication

I. Strong, Michelle, author

II. Milton, Nancy Lee, author

Your Weight Loss G-Spot :

The Woman's How-To Weight Loss System For A Healthy, Sassy You!

Michelle Strong, Nancy Milton.

Issued in print and electronic formats.

ISBN 978-0-9940408-8-6 (bound)

ISBN 978-0-9940408-7-9 (paperback)

ISBN 978-0-9940408-6-2 (epub)

ISBN 978-0-9940408-4-8 (pdf)

ISBN 978-0-9940408-5-5 (kindle)

ISBN 978-0-9940408-9-3 (kobo)

1. Weight loss.
2. Reducing diets.
3. Women--Nutrition.
4. Women--Health and hygiene.

RM222.2.S78 2015

613.2'5082

C2015-907952-7

DEDICATION

For my mom. The unconditional care and support you show me on a daily basis is overwhelming. Thank you for loving me so profoundly.

To my husband Blake. You bring "ying" to my crazy "yang" - thank you for your patience, encouragement and for being the voice of reason. You are amazing, I love you.

To my friends and family who cheer me on, you mean the world to me.

Xo

Michelle

To you:

The gal with the courage and charged tenacity to figure this "weight crap" out, once and for all.

Sister, it's time to "clean house" and I'm with you every step.

You deserve this.

With love and gratitude

Nance xo

ENDORSEMENTS

An inventive approach to self-help, weight-loss and healing that is practical, educational and inspirational. A must read!

-Dr. C. Christoforou ND

Your Weight Loss G-Spot sizzles with a brave energy! As a Fitness Professional for over 25 years, this book is a must read. "Your Weight Loss G-Spot" will be my go-to-guide for many years to come because of its mind-body approach that is often lacking in the fitness and health industry. It inspires the reader to have a deeper awareness of their thoughts and feelings towards why and what they eat. The authors were able to take a difficult topic and turn it into a current, compelling, humorous read that I will be recommending to all of my fitness professional colleagues and clients.

-Julie Henderson-Young, Group Fitness Divisional Manager - Goodlife Fitness Clubs

Most diet books just tell you what to eat. Your Weight Loss G-Spot is refreshingly different. This book offers you proven tools and a system which is designed to help you stick to your diet. After all, when and how you eat is just as important as what you eat. And the fact that the authors are playfully and candidly connecting nutrition to sex on just about every other page, keeps you reading and engaged. If you have ever struggled with weight gain, inability to stay on track or no willpower, then this book is for you.

-Igor Klibanov, Author, STOP EXERCISING! The Way You Are Doing it Now.

Nancy and Michelle, with their collective expertise, introduce a new position to assist women in their weight loss struggle.

-Antonella Morra MD

Michelle and Nancy bring the lessons of personal experience, cover the fundamentals of healthy nutrition, provide some tasty "food for thought" and delight with a palette of beautiful and delicious recipes. This book will not only feed your brain with knowledge of health, but also nourish your soul with humour and the heartfelt wisdom of two women who get it.

-Sita Kacker, co-owner Power Yoga Canada Georgetown

Can't really speak to the G-spot question. Out of my depth on that one. But I can say that if you want a smart, useful and practical approach to not only getting leaner and healthier, but also understanding why, this book will work for you."

-Damien Cox, Sports broadcaster, journalist and author

I am so unbelievably excited for the release of "Your Weight Loss G-Spot", not so much for myself per se, but it is a fun and factual spin on the main topics health professionals combat daily with their clients. As a personal trainer, many of my clients are females between the ages of 30-60, and I think that this book will absolutely be the difference maker to them, especially topics that a male trainer often can have difficulty discussing with their female clients.

Knowing and working with Michelle for the past six years, I am not surprised that this book highlights all of the key misconceptions, concepts and strategies we have utilized with all of our clients. Having seen the amazing results she is able to produce, (my own mother being one of them) I know that the advice that she has spelled out in this book will truly make the difference in the readers' life.

The principles they have laid out in the book have been proven time and time again with their own clients. In one section the authors mention Jack Canfield's "The Success Principles," a book I am currently reading, and I think it is important to emphasis Jack's key phrase "The principles always work if you always work on the principles," because if you follow the guidance of Nancy and Michelle, I can certainly guarantee success!

Congratulations ladies, this truly is a fantastic read!

-Rory Kosonic CPT, CSCS

A brilliant and inventive approach to self-help, weight-loss and positive lifestyle change from two authors who have helped countless people change their lives.

-Dr. T. Nahirny MD

Your Weight Loss G-Spot is mind-blowing and disruptive to some long-standing beliefs about what our bodies require for optimal health. This book contains the definitive weight loss system and no-nonsense approach to win against the familiar internal voices that keep us from becoming our best self. Michelle and Nancy have got you covered with expert coaching, easy to follow examples and plans, powerful tools that work and a healthy dose of humour to help you implement and achieve your goals!

-François Beauregard, World Muscle Model Champion, Drug-Free Athlete

ACKNOWLEDGEMENTS

The culminations of many people have gone into helping get this book to where it is today- without this support, these last three years wouldn't have been possible.

Thank you to my clients who have shared their health stories with me. Without knowing it, you have contributed greatly to my professional growth.

A huge thank you to Nicole Lem, photographer extraordinaire! You captured a beautifully simple, light-hearted shot for our cover.

To those who helped produce this book, Dieter, Kristy and teams, thank you.

To my co-writer Nancy, I knew nine years ago when we met it would be the start of a great bond. Thank you for your wisdom and friendship.

For my family and friends, thank you for your confidence. Daily I can feel your support and encouragement, which has given me the drive to keep pushing. I love you to the moon and back.

Xo

Michelle

FOREWORD

When Michelle told me that she had written a book called the "Your Weight Loss G- Spot" I was immediately intrigued. What a fantastic catchy title. I was excited to read this book myself so I can tell my patients. Once I began reading the book, I was so captivated and entertained with the writing style and humour that I was unable to put it down. I was hooked!

Michelle and originally I connected as natural healers in the industry. She was searching for a Naturopathic Doctor in the Oakville/Mississauga area to whom she can refer patients for stress management beyond nutrition. Based on her own personal experience with acupuncture, Michelle was seeking a Naturopathic Doctor that used acupuncture for stress management. I was a perfect fit for her as I deal with many patients suffering from stress and frequently use acupuncture and other wonderful modalities (such as B12 injections, supplements and IV therapy) to treat them. At the same time, I was looking for a holistic nutritionist who can sit down with my patients and give them step-by-step recipes and plans to achieve their health goals. As a busy Naturopathic Doctor, sometimes it is extremely time consuming going through step-by-step recipes for patients. We normally just tell our patients to follow a hypoallergenic diet or an anti-inflammatory diet. We would give them hand outs and printed recipes only and have them read and follow them. I knew that by sending my patients to Michelle, she would give them that extra time to go through the dietary changes step-by-step.

As soon as Michelle and I met up we hit it off immediately. It felt like I was talking to another me, someone who was passionate and excited about health and helping patients as I was.

We immediately began referring patients back and forth to one another and e-mailing each other to exchange our expertise and ideas on how to further assist our patients. It was the beginning of a wonderful relationship.

I have been a Naturopathic Doctor serving the Mississauga area for almost 10 years. I opened the doors to my clinic, the Holistix Naturopathic Health Clinic, back in 2006. Over the years, the Holistix team has managed to stay on top by receiving the Readers Choice Award for the best Naturopathic Clinic in Mississauga from 2008 until present (2015). We have also won the Top Choice Award in Mississauga for the best Alternative Clinic in 2012 and the best Holistic Healthcare Clinic in 2013. We always strive in providing the best naturopathic care for our patients.

Both Michelle and Nancy have taken a whole new spin on achieving your weight loss goals that are easy to follow. I find that most of my patients do need encouragement for weight loss, not only by making the right food choices but adapting to a style and sticking to it!! What I found intriguing in this book is that it really does feel that both Michelle and Nancy are right beside you, helping you along the way. The thought-provoking activities, quizzes and relaxation exercises make this book feel like an interactive manual with someone right there to make you laugh and help you along the way when you are feeling down, reminding you that it is all worthwhile. Both Michelle and Nancy are brilliant at making the parallels to sex. They manage to take a bland topic and spice it up with witty innuendoes. They focus on encouragement, support and having a vision and sticking to it by reminding yourself of the vision and owning up to your failures.

I have read various books to help patients with their journey of reaching their weight loss goals and I would find it hard to finish the book. For the first time, we have a weight loss book that is easy to read, informative, interactive, educational and hilarious!! Why not make weight loss fun? Having both a holistic nutritionist and life coach to help you along the way is ideal to achieving your weight loss goals. How do we keep everyone interested? Start talking about sex? Genius! A must read that will allow anyone to achieve their weight loss goals. I will definitely be referring my patients to this book. I am confident that they will be ecstatic with their success and that they will be referring this book to family and friends. I know I will!!

Dr. Christina Christoforou B.Sc. Hons., N.D.

Naturopathic Doctor/Owner

Holistix Naturopathic Health Clinic

www.holistixclinic.com

HOW TO USE THIS BOOK

Your Weight Loss G-Spot is a make-it-happen weight loss book that combines the fundamentals of nutrition and healthy eating with the mind–body–emotion targeted coaching required to get you to your goal and to make it stick.

Michelle Strong (BA, RHN), your nutritionist will lay out a clear plan to prepare both your kitchen and your stomach for weight loss success.

Nancy your Certified Coach and International Intention Speaker (CPCC, ACC, PCC) will get real with coaching exercises and techniques to help you take control and shift your beliefs on you and food as you view it today.

Chapter by chapter, Michelle will guide you through the ins and outs of a hands-on weight loss program and Nancy will offer insight and support for the emotional journey that accompanies this process.

This is not a "get skinny quick" book; Your Weight Loss G-Spot provides a realistic approach that has proven successful over and over again with our clients.

What you need: a pen or pencil, the free workbook that you can download below and the right frame of mind. We dare you to step into the beginning of the rest of your life!

Xo

Michelle and Nancy

FREE BOOK UPDATES, VIDEOS AND RESOURCES

Want to learn more? We have created a free workbook to go along with this book. You will also find a list of great documentaries, books, websites and other valuable bonus resources to will help you dive deeper!

Get access to your free bonus resources at

http://bonus.weightlossgspot.com/

Table of Contents

1

FALLING IN LUST WITH YOUR DIET

Hi! It's Nancy here, your Mind Body Spirit Guru and 'Get Real' Coach. Ready to get started?

Let's do this!

"Oh, look! Yet another book about losing weight," your petulant inner voice says. "Next!"

"Screw you, inner voice," revolts your more mature, wiser self. "This time, it's different. This time, it's about me, for me, within me…"

"Watch me!"

If your voice—the voice of your real, authentic self—has brought you to this book then yaaaaaaaay! We are ready for you. In fact, you choosing this book also means that YOU are ready for you.

It's time to find Your Weight Loss G-Spot once and for all!

Yes, I said it…

G-Spot

G-Spot G-Spot G-Spot

Doesn't that feel sooooo good to say—over and over and over?

Let's be clear: there are many things in life we all desire, and the list looks different for everyone. You may strive for a great education, true love, a fulfilling career, passion, happiness, family, lots of vacation time, a huge, magical, super organized walk-in closet... the list goes on and on.

But there are two wants that consistently arise at the Ladies Only Table: weight loss and better sex. It's true. And while I have no trouble at all talking about either subject, I'd love it if we were all this comfortable! If you wish the same, this book is for you!

Because what woman doesn't want to know how to best activate her G-Spot and weight loss?

Abracadabra! Here you go!

When it comes to getting down and dirty, you and I both know that no two bodies are exactly the same. You need to be intimately aware of your parts to find out what makes you tick, what enables your body to reach its peak level, your triggers and your pleasure points, etc.

This book "thinks" along those same lines. Because we are all completely unique, for this plan to work (from reading, to applying, to results), you need to be involved and invested. This means dedicating yourself to a vision and creating a consequence for yourself if you don't complete an action—or a reward when you do. YOU'RE calling the shots.

Why? Simple!

Because you are in charge of you. Only you can do this for yourself. This book is going to teach you how to take charge of being healthy, making good-for-you decisions and standing tall and proud in the lifestyle you want to have. Whatever speed bump has slowed you down in the past—

even if it's been five years of hitting speed bump after speed bump—it's time to steamroll right over them!

Because there is always a choice. Sometimes people get stuck in "stuff" and they think there is no way out. We disagree! There is always a way—or ways—out and sometimes these ways are HARD, but there is always a choice to be made. You choosing how you use this book is one of those choices. Use it like the Yellow Pages, a journal, a textbook or your Bible. There are many, completely different approaches to taking in the content and then applying it. It's your journey; therefore, it's your choice.

Because we all have different timelines. Some of you want this, like, yesterday and are looking to sprint to the finish line. Others have been battling for 30 years and are prepared to adopt a more slow and steady wins the race approach. And others would simply be keen to learn five key tips that will influence better decisions for their life, both short and long term. It's your clock. It's your time. Your race. Your life. We are here as a supportive resource and different from anything else you have tried. And part of the reason we're different is that if you agree to commit to this, there is no try. Nope. You have a choice to make right now: either "I'm going to do it," OR "I'm going to try to do it." Who do you want to be? MMMHmmm. Thought so. This book isn't about TRYing.

It's about DOing, which will bring you to actually BEing the change.

This workbook is going to push you. It's going to (re)teach you how to push yourself. You are going to (re)connect with accountability to your health, your lifestyle, and your choices. Some days you are going to loathe the book. And that's okay. We can handle it. As long as you're willing to work through the discomfort, you'll discover the magic waiting for you on the other side.

This book will help you uncover stuff you didn't even know was in your way. It will also help you dig out what you've buried because you didn't know it was in your way. And the book is going to give you amazing, healthy, EASY tips and tricks to make this a life-changer.

That's it.

That's the concept.

Excited? This is just the beginning!

Now, just so we're clear, we've never seen a Chapter 1 (a) and (b) in any book, either, but knowing how seldom the prologue and introduction of a book actually get read, we needed to make sure we're all on the same page. Are we there? If so, let's move on to the other Chapter 1—Chapter 1 (b).

CHAPTER 1 (B) FOREPLAY

In Rodgers and Hammerstein's The Sound of Music, Maria sang: "Let's start at the very beginning; a very good place to start..."

We agree with Maria for a number of solid reasons. Consider this: would you prefer to start at the beginning, in the middle or close to the end?

Depends on what you're starting! Personally, I would prefer starting at the beginning for the majority of things: a movie, a good book, a vacation, a friendship, a new car and of course, sex (duh—isn't foreplay the precursor to awesome sex?). Actually, come to think of it, other than housekeeping or eating a meal (which I'd prefer to begin with dessert), I am definitely a start-at-the-beginning gal. And specifically for this life project you're about to embrace, there are lots of reasons we need to begin at the beginning with you.

Starting at the beginning will allow you to get clear on how you got Here in the first place.

What is Here?

Well, it's different for every one of us but we're assuming your Here isn't the healthiest, happiest place. Here are several reasons why you may now find yourself Here, despite your best intentions:

Yoyo dieting

Poor portion management

Sugar addiction

Salt cravings

Poor food choices

Little or no meal planning

Emotional eating

Thoughts like: "Exercise sucks," "Once I start eating, I can't stop," "I've lost control," "I've never had control," "I manage my weight with physical activity only," etc.

Do any of these resonate with you?

Fact is, how you got Here could be due to one of the factors above, or a combination of many. But it's your Here that we, right now, want to pinpoint and own... then drop like a hot potato. You making it your scapegoat ain't helping your situation!

So let's make like Maria and start at the very beginning of what you consider your journey with food. Why are we doing this again?

To gain insight into essential information, like your relationship with food, the role food has played in your life to date, what and how you are influenced, habits you hold and boundaries that may be holding you back. Looking at your starting point and, potentially more important, your additional turning points, will allow us to better create a plan to get you where you want to be, making your past experiences "learning" versus triggers or barriers.

Reflection is an amazing life tool because it can provide stepping stones to another path you can take, versus repeatedly taking the same path you keep tripping on. Often we think we are reflecting, but instead we're simply rehashing. The difference? Rehashing is repeating the same story in your head again and again. The story plays in your head like a song on repeat. Ironically, this story you've created actually does you way more harm than good (and you'll learn more about this when you get to Michelle's chapter on stress). You repeat the story enough times and it can start to define you. Let's do the reverse instead: find and repeat the positives, the key behaviours and inspirations, and view other ways we can see our situation.

Instead of repeating, let's reflect, with some powerful questions that will allow us to be clear on what's working for you and what's not. We'll find out where the gaps are, and then design a better, customized plan that works for YOU, based on YOU.

Clearing

We all have a story. Some people are positively powered by their history. For others, their past sits neutrally within them. They have moved on and continued to have other experiences. For some of us, though, our story holds us hostage, and we can't figure out why. We know we want to change the holding pattern but we're unaware of what it is, or that we're even in one!

So what does the term 'clearing' mean? I define the term 'clearing' as making the space in your head, and in your heart, to see and feel differently. For example, if you were clearing a plot of land, you might clear trees (roots included), remove bushes and overgrown stuff and end up with an open space. You might use this new space for something different, something awesome. You writing out your story is like clearing the space for you to write a new one for yourself, versus constantly repeating the one that's clearly not working for you. WOW! Imagine the power that would give you!

That's why, for us, for you, you need to get your story down on paper. It's guaranteed to give you release, freedom, clarity and awareness. So worth it!

If you haven't done anything like this before, be prepared for some strong emotions to rise within you: anxiousness, unease, hesitation, vulnerability, feeling pushed out of your comfort zone, fear of what you may find. Take a deep breath and whatever feeling comes up, just BE with it.

Why? It's time. You bought this book for a reason. YOU. Yep. You want change. You want better for yourself. You want your Here to be different.

Different is good! Different is going to give you something you haven't found for yourself yet. That's why you're here with us. We're doing this together. If it doesn't feel different, it's not going to work.

So, step one. Write your story. But what should you write? Here are some basic parameters; the rest is up to you.

Think about your history. Your upbringing, home life, school life, work life, interests and influences for health and wellness, plus food milestones. How did you learn about food? How did your parents act around food and feel about food? Was it used in times of celebration or in times of sadness? What feelings were connected to it? What impact did it have? Whatever comes up, write it down.

The only rules are these:

- Your story can be any length.

- Find a way to enjoy the process by finding a comfy, neutral place to sit and reflect.

- Give yourself a window of time.

- And write! Because the last rule is, you can't pick up this book again until you've completed this exercise.

I know. We're sticklers. But you want to get this right! These parameters are designed for your success.

Still unsure where to begin? Jump, girl! You bought this book to get real with your Here. Half the time we aren't having better sex and climaxing because we're thinking too much. You're pulling the same thing here. Get out of your head and write from your heart. Your heart needs to be explored, your feelings need to be named and acknowledged so we know what we're working with in order to move forward. Connecting with your heart will help get you the results you want. Stop thinking and start writing. 3-2-1 GO!

Let me give you a full-on nudge by providing a template. Just fill in the blanks in your workbook!

You can find this exercise in the workbook!

=>> http://bonus.weightlossgspot.com

My Food Story

By _____. Here's what I know:

_____

_____

_____

Ta-da! Step one completed. That might have been easy for you, or it might have taken three weeks. Either way, you've done it. Way to go! Now what?

Our next step is to reread what you have written while considering the following terms: Enabler, Inhibitor, Excuses, Mindset Shifts and Root Cause(s). First, we need to agree on what each term means and how it impacts you. In our words, here are the definitions.

Enabler: Something or someone that is making it easy for you to stay where you are (stuck!) in your journey to move away from your Here. Example: "In my culture, everything revolves around eating together and sharing meals."

Inhibitor: An inhibitor is actually holding you back from moving from your Here. The difference between an enabler and an inhibitor is that an enabler is often camouflaged as positive, whereas an inhibitor is seen as a negative. Example: "My mom has always said I'm big-boned."

Excuses: These are things you tell yourself or others about why you are where you are with your Here. Examples include: "I work too many hours to make time for myself," "My family is my top priority right

now," "I'll start Monday," "I'll start after just one more
_____ (cookie, plateful, helping, etc.)"

Mindset: Mindset acknowledges the way you see your situation. It's your approach or perspective. Examples include: "My whole family is heavy, it's just my genetic makeup," "I've tried everything! This is hopeless."

Root cause: The four definitions listed above are things that are getting in your way of moving forward from your Here. The root cause of the situation sheds light on why you are doing or not doing what is the best decision for you. Knowing the root cause will help create a concrete action plan to move forward. Example: "From re-reading my food story I can see the theme that I have created with food," "I don't deal with my emotions and I eat through them instead of dealing with them fully."

With those informal definitions outlined, using coloured highlighters or some kind of labelling system, reread your story and identify some key reasons for your Here in your past. For example:

Enablers = blue

Inhibitors = purple

Excuses = orange

Mindset shifts = pink

Root cause = green

Now is not the time to hesitate. You want to find your G-Spot? Grab a flashlight (a.k.a. your trusty highlighter) and start looking. Your treasure map is right in front of you!

When you are done highlighting your story, keep reading – starting from here.

Are you back? Good!

Let's recap to make sure we're at the same place:

Have you:

Written your food story?

Highlighted your story, noting various themes?

The next step is to reflect on what you have recorded, by answering the following questions in as much detail as you need.

But wait! Before you start…

When I say reflect, I don't mean just going through the motions. I mean you should feel something deep down in your gut, a major shift in your perspective or view.

This is a game-changing moment. An "Oh my gosh, I just realized _____." When you get to this aha! moment, congratulations. You're one step closer to Your Weight Loss G-Spot.

Now, ask yourself honestly:

What was your biggest surprise when you reviewed your story?

_____

_____

_____

Describe what was toughest for you to record about your story.

_____

_____

_____

What emotions are attached to it? (This could be any emotion: anger, frustration, feeling flustered, feeling "found out," embarrassed, sad, lighter, a sense of relief, etc.)

_____

_____

_____

Looking at the coding system for the themes you found in your story, which one is most keeping you in the plateau of Here? What colour pops up the most often? Is it enabler, inhibitor, excuses, mindset?

Record in your workbook specifically how this is impacting your approach to moving forward in your life.

_____

_____

_____

Here's some insight for you, depending what you uncovered in this exercise.

Excuse driven

If you discovered that your story's primary theme was excuse-driven, our suggestions while reading this book include:

- Be aware of how quickly your instinct tells you to ignore an exercise, a chapter or the book entirely.

- Know that it takes 21 days minimum to create a NEW habit. Be fair to yourself here! You need to unwind the bad habit (i.e. creating an excuse) before you can begin the new habit. Give yourself 60 days before you label this a failure.

Take on SMALL bites that are easier to digest, leading to QUICKER wins that amp up your motivation level. If you're a bit of a gobbler like me, the definition of a small bite is something that is doable. It's the equivalent to a step towards your goal habit, versus an unbalanced, fingers crossed, "hope I get it this time" leap. To recap: ANYTHING you do to change a habit and create a new one needs to be small enough to be easily achievable. You know this about yourself. If you make it too large, too soon, it feels unobtainable and you'll quit, feeling worse than ever.

Find someone you can count on to be accountable to throughout this process. What will this look like? What can he or she say to you when you start with excuses?

The moment you start forming an excuse in your head, pause and ask yourself, "what's the real reason?" because this lame excuse isn't it!

My guess is that you're the excuse! Time to suck it up, sweetheart. You want Your Weight Loss G-Spot? You've got to lose the excuses—and that starts in that moment.

Inhibitor driven

If your story theme was primarily inhibitor-driven, here are some areas for you to consider:

Think about a positive influence and/or role model in your life. How can you better utilize that relationship to support you through this life-changing experience?

Consider a different approach to handling the inhibitors in your life. This could include spending less time with them and filtering what they say by how you interpret their words, tone and/or body language.

Create your own armour to protect yourself from how the inhibitor(s) currently impact you. If your inhibitor is a something versus a someone, using a blank piece of paper, record the something in the middle of the page. Now circle it and draw eight short lines starting from that circle. At the end of each line, record something that is the opposite of what's in the circle. Choose one you like the most. Own it (and cross out the lame inhibitor in the centre, because you just released it from yourself for life)!

Enabler driven

If your primary story theme was enabler-driven, here are some areas for you to consider:

Get clear on how your enabler(s) mean well by the way they are currently supporting you in your life.

Consider what tweaks need to be made to better support/cheerlead to help you reach your Here.

Objectively, what parameters will you ask for and also offer them, to make this journey better for you both, and in the end, improve your relationship? If your enabler was a statement or thing that granted you permission to act in this fashion, write the thing or statement on a blank piece of paper. Now put the paper through the shredder, burn it in a fire pit outside, crumple it into a ball and toss it away. YOU get to choose! Choose to control your own thoughts and stop the insanity of living the statement that someone else labelled you with!

Mindset driven

Finally, if your story theme was mostly Mindset-Driven, consider areas in your life that you confidently own. What's different about your mindset or approach on those tasks or projects, versus your mindset on your Here?

How is self-talk getting in the way of your positive approach? Or maybe the better question: knowing you have full control over the thoughts in your head and can choose what those thoughts are, what five thoughts (write them down now) would be better options for you to repeat in your head versus the current ones you are using?

Lastly, we are more successful with self-accountability when we are emotionally connected to our goal. Specific to weight loss, what's your emotional tie to losing the pounds? Whatever the reason, if it is without a heart-felt connection to you, there is a large chance you won't pull this off. A goal without passion is like a car without gas in the tank or a vibrator without batteries – you'll get nowhere fast. The question for you to answer is what makes this important to me in my head and my heart?

_____

_____

_____

Summary

To recap:

We all have a beginning. This is where we all got started. And we've all made missteps along the way.

But congratulations! You just explored, in detail, how your beginning plays a role in why you have picked up this book. You now have insight on some of the reasons you are where you are!

Here's the good news. Every day is a new beginning. As Deepak Chopra says, "The past is history, the future is a mystery, and this moment is a gift. That's why this moment is called the present."

Time to open your gift!

Take and use this knowledge of where you're currently faltering in your health journey to adjust and get what you want.

As Dr. Seuss says in his book, _Oh, The Places You'll Go!_:

Congratulations, today is your day

You're off to great places you're off and away

You have brains in your head and feet in your shoes

And no one chooses the direction for you, but you…"

So. This is it. Play or pass. Time to choose. Now is the starting line for a new day or you can repeat your old patterns of behaviour and get the same results.

Ask yourself this:

From the journaling you did above, what are TWO specific things you will do from this moment forward to make things better for yourself in your health quest?

Your beliefs are your actions. Rewrite the label-free story you need, that will from now forward be the story you recite in your heart and your head, that will get you and keep you where you want to be.

_____

_____

_____

Thinking ahead: In Chapter 4, we get intimate in your kitchen. Knowing this now, you can begin to think about the food products that you know aren't G-Spot friendly foods. We tell you this now so when it's kitchen purge time, you don't have a meltdown! We have a purge system that works and we don't want you to be surprised. Get started today. And let's be honest—we know that you know (for the most part) which items aren't really food!

Chapter 1: Keys to G

- Take the time to understand first what has gotten in your way from finding Your Weight Loss G-Spot, and then release those barriers for today, and your future. This release can be like a flashlight in a dark tunnel of the G-Spot quest...

- Remember, you have choice. You always have choice. Some choices may seem harder than others in the moment, but you get to choose you.

2

BUT I WANT THE UNICORN WITH THE BIG HORN!

Nancy here. Time to get clear on our goals!

I love how our minds spin. We're so creative! So imaginative! Consider the scenarios we conjure up based on absolutely zero evidence!

There can be a beauty to this—but there can also be crazy-making pain, depending what shape we allow our thoughts to take.

When it comes to weight loss, often the ideas we spin in our heads are a combination of these extremes. We have this vision of ourselves at a certain weight/size/shape that seems almost unattainable, yet in this insane vision, we somehow get there while still eating the unhealthy foods we crave.

Sounds ideal, right?

But then we start "The Program" (cue horror movie sound effects). It's Day One and we're now at the other extreme of our vision. We feel starved, depleted, empty. Why is this so hard, we wonder? How come other people can do this and I fail? In your head, you envision your poor tummy, with nary a crumb to satiate your hunger. You're wasting away to nothing… and it's only noon!

Is any of this ringing a bell? Or perhaps a gong?

Dreaming and visioning as a practice can be very impactful and, if utilized well, can bring WOWie results. But an unhealthy vision will bring you nothing but misery. We, of course, are in full support of helping you create a healthy vision. This chapter will show you how using the Your Weight Loss G-Spot approach.

Let me tell you a story I call "The Finish Line."

When I was 21, I ran my first and only full marathon. A marathon is 42.6 kilometres or 26 miles. I started training more than four months ahead of race day, adding two km a week until I got to 26 km. I had read somewhere that, for full marathon preparation, training just shy of the full distance was ideal, because you'd be close enough to the distance that on race day, you'd find your stride, slip into the runners' zone and your adrenaline would get you to the finish line.

Sounds easy enough, right?

Race day was scheduled for mid-October; in Toronto, Canada, this could mean we could expect any kind of weather. Well, Mother Nature decided to pull out all the stops: we got sun, we got rain, it was overcast, we had hail, we had wind… and that combination repeated itself all day.

I was young. At the starting line, my stomach churned like I'd been on the Tilt-A-Whirl for an hour blindfolded. My heart dropped like it had when I was a kid, lost in the shopping mall. And my head spun with a kazillion thoughts, all relating to my running skill level, my focus and where I fit within this world of endurance. We were crammed like sardines behind the starting line, jumpy and jittery, waiting to begin. The starter shot the gun and the longest run of my life began.

You name the emotion, I felt it that day. WOWie highs of pride and the thrill of the chase. And lows that included the certainty that my body would never feel this bad again.

About 8 kilometres from the finish line, I kept looking down at my legs because my knees were aching so much I thought my bones were protruding from them. I'm sure I was starting to hallucinate.

Then, something happened. From somewhere deep inside my consciousness, a vision I had used during my training—an image of a red finish line—came into my mind, rippling lightly in the breeze and pulling me towards it.

For the next 7.75 kilometres, that's all I saw. Not the police manning the crowds, not the road barriers, not the well-wishers holding up their handmade signs and ringing their cow bells, not even the runners passing me. It was just me and my vision of that tattered red finish line.

I had never run a marathon before. Clearly, this vision was one my mind gifted me when I needed it most. And guess what?

It worked. With 0.25 km left, I saw the real finish line. With a combination of joy and pain, through tears and a triumphant grin, I completed my first and last marathon.

The reason I share this story is to inspire you to question your current vision skills and compare them with what they could be.

My guess is that your visioning skills are at a beginner level, like mine were, and therefore you're not reaching your best potential. Reflecting on my story, it's clear that somehow, close to the end of the race, something kicked in and granted me the finish line vision. I'm darn fortunate that it happened, too. It's what powered me to complete the challenge.

But look at all of the missed opportunities for visioning that would have set me up for a way better race day mindset.

A clear vision could have been a crucial touchstone during the race and provided me with an emotional connection to help me reach my goal.

We—you and me, working together—need to tap into this power to create Your Weight Loss G-Spot vision. So grab a pen and your trusty workbook and let's get going!

Step One: Start With Your Finish Line In Mind

Describe, using as much detail as possible, what your own finish line looks like. Include colours, textures, scents and sights. What does it feel like here? What senses do you feel firing? Close your eyes and imagine what this looks like. Where are you? What are you wearing? What colour are your clothes? How does your body feel? Record how you feel when you walk and when you talk. What's your outlook on life?

_____

_____

_____

Step Two: Ask Yourself—What's In It For Me?

When I facilitate sessions on how to explain things so a listener connects with the content, I talk about features and benefits.

Features "tell" about the product or service you're trying to promote, while benefits "sell" how that product or service will make life better or easier. Benefits are customized to the individual. This is key! For anyone to really buy into an idea, product or service, it needs to resonate personally with them.

Let's use the example of buying a house. You're looking for a home with a large, renovated kitchen. That's a feature. The benefits of this feature for you might be: lots of cupboard space, more room for kitchen parties, a big counter space to prep food, modern, well-equipped and tastefully decorated and there's room for family meals, which you consider important to stay connected.

Bottom line: a benefit isn't a benefit unless it resonates with the person you're communicating with. It's imperative that you're crystal clear about why your finish line vision resonates with you. This and only this will make you focus on it, stick to it and with it, and follow through.

This must land with you in order for you to commit fully to it!

Ask yourself, "Why do I want this?" Ask it over and over until you get to the real root of the reason.

Using the table below, list both the features and benefits of your finish line vision. Try to come up with multiple benefits under each feature.

FEATURE	BENEFIT

For example:

FEATURE	BENEFITS
A PROPORTIONATE HIP TO BELLY RATIO	✓ Jeans that fit like they were made for me ✓ The ability to move comfortably within my body shape ✓ Feeling confident in my skin ✓ Being able to get up from a seated position and not having to adjust my shirt over my body like a drop cloth
FEEL CONFIDENT IN MY BODY	✓ The ease to move more lightly with every step ✓ Convey the strength I feel in other aspects of my life with how I look ✓ My inner presence helps me to connect faster and easier with others
PREVENTIVE HEALTH; I.E. TO BE AROUND FOR MY KIDS AND GRANDKIDS	✓ Better food choices, therefore better energy levels ✓ I'll sleep more soundly
SIZE X JEANS	✓ I'll feel sexy and reignite my sex life

To complete this exercise, review your list and circle which benefit and which feature resonates most with you.

Step Three: Spot The Unicorn

First, read what you recorded for Step One. Then review the key benefit you circled in Step Two.

Time to get real. Is the visual you imagined in Step One believable to you?

When I use the term "spot the unicorn", that means it's time to get the unrealistic, not-gonna-happen-ever stuff out of your vision.

Why? Because if you don't think it's doable now, how the heck are you going to make it when you're depending on your vision to get you through a rough patch or a tough day?

Just so we're on the same page, I'll share with you my finish line. First, read my brief history so you'll have some background information. Keeping in mind that my vision needs to work for me, read the following versions of my finish line and compare them.

Brief History

Client: Nancy

Age: 42

Height: 5'10"

Weight: 160 lb.

Activity level: Intense: 6 to 10 times per week

The Real Story: Nancy is a real rules-oriented gal. She's never tried coffee, smoking or drugs—but cookies and ice cream are like kryptonite for her! Her meals are either very healthy or cuckoo sweet. Eating in moderation is a challenge for her every day.

Version One: Nancy's Finish Line Vision

I'm at home, in my kitchen. I'm 35 lbs. lighter than my typical weight. I'm wearing a pair of jeans that fit me like a dream, like they were made for me, yet I can comfortably breathe and move. I feel like a runway model. I am muffin-top free. The muscles I have developed from my years of activity are now clearly visible because they are no longer covered with excess fat. I am super healthy. I am super energetic. I am super vibrant. I eat a full breakfast, lunch and dinner. I never yearn for desserts. I am easily satisfied with snacks that include a handful of almonds or an apple with almond butter. This feels easy.

Version Two: Nancy's Finish Line Vision

I'm at home, in my kitchen. I feel settled. Settled in my own skin. The daily haunting of what I'm eating is no longer with me. My body and I have come to an agreement (yes, sometimes for me they did feel like two separate things), and we're on comfortable parameters for eating and activity that I can live with feeling happy and centered versus restricted and missing out. I am ten pounds lighter than my typical weight. I move comfortably in my clothing and in my body. I am healthy. I am energetic. I am vibrant. The pressure of thinking "maybe today, I'll start," is gone. Today is here and I've got this! It's just part of me now.

What similarities did you spot? In both versions, there's a sense of success, a feeling of "I've got this." The healthy, energetic and vibrant me reside in both. And in both, the vision takes place in my own kitchen—where the food is!

What differences did you spot? To me, there's an ease in the tone of Version Two that speaks to goals that are realistic and achievable. The language of Version Two suggests that thought and consideration has been put into food and lifestyle based on goals. Version Two demonstrates that the head and the heart have joined up to make a conscious decision about long-term changes that will provide a better life without feeling stretched and missing out.

Did you spot the unicorn in Version One? It's the finish line for the grapefruit diet (do you remember this impossible diet plan?), otherwise known as unrealistic.

It's about behaviour change but I don't hear the belief behind the change, which means there is a large chance of it being short-lived.

How can you spot this? Consider how dreamlike it seems. It's missing the realistic piece: a weight loss that's actually achievable. For example, I couldn't weigh 125 pounds at this height. And come on, really? I am 42 years old and not aspiring to be a Victoria's Secret model.

Yet this weight, this size, this bully-like expectation of the impossible is where we often go first when we set goals. How's that for setting yourself up for failure?

So Now It's Your Turn!

From what you listed in Steps One and Two, draft two versions for yourself for your finish line vision. Make one as close to what you've always created in your head, ever since you first started the weight loss game. Create Version Two after reviewing Version One. Include the benefits that you circled in Step Two. Incorporate details that suit both versions. Acknowledge the "unicorn" in your story and what's realistic for today and tomorrow. Be fair to yourself.

It's time.

Version One:

_____

_____

_____

Version Two:

_____

_____

_____

And ta da! You've now got a vision for yourself! My advice here? Take a breather. Finish this paragraph and close the book for the rest of the day. Acknowledge the really big step you just took. You just stepped into your big-girl, "I own this" pants. You just got real with yourself. Good for you!

And welcome back!

After that great written vision exercise, it's time to develop a physical replica. In my industry, we call this a vision board.

Envision It!

"Action without vision is only passing time, vision without action is merely daydreaming, but vision with action can change the world."

~ Nelson Mandela

No wonder Nelson Mandela won the hearts of millions with his inspiring way of looking at the world. He had an incredible ability to demonstrate the need to take action instead of sitting around waiting for things to happen. Some people are naturally blessed with this gift: to see beyond themselves to navigate life with supreme purpose, and then take action on their beliefs.

Most of us need a little shove in the right direction! If that's you, you're not alone. But hallelujah! We have a simple solution.

A vision board is a tool that's very effective in helping clarify a goal. Through words and pictures, the story of your ambitions, your aspirations and your desires are brought to life.

It's a collection of all your goals assembled together for the sole purpose of a) literally forcing you to identity your goals and b) reminding you and reinforcing these goals on a daily basis. Both of these concepts are super important. We have already learned how important it is to clarify your finish line for Your Weight Loss G-Spot goal, but what does this actually look like on a vision board?

Dream It, Live It

There are many different ways to create your own vision board.

> **Tip:** Try Oprah's O Dreamboard. You need to be a member of Oprah.com to access this, but it only takes a few minutes, it's free and you have everything you need right there to start creating. Simply search "O Dreamboard" on her site (www.oprah.com) and you'll be led, step-by-step, to create your own stunning virtual vision board.

The old-school method is tried and true: just grab a Bristol board, some inspiring magazine pictures, glue and scissors and start cutting and pasting. If you're feeling extra-crafty, head to your local art store and grab some cool paper, stickers and markers.

Or, for you super-savvy, more technologically advanced folks, create a vision board online using programs like Pinterest. There is no right way... just your way!

When I created my current vision board, I asked a magazine-loving friend for a pile of used editions that I could cut up. I took an hour one Sunday afternoon and pulled pages from the magazine, focusing on what made my heart lift when I saw the picture, word or image. I cut them out and put them in a file.

A week later, I went back to the file and culled the pictures. I kept those I still connected with and attached them to my vision board. I added some family pictures and a sentence I have written about living authentically.

What to keep in mind when designing you vision board:

- Your goal

- A timeline you've decided on for your specific goal; e.g. six months or a year

- Remember to feel your way through this exercise (versus thinking your way through it)

- Think BIG and only choose images that get your juices flowing

- Don't worry about anybody else. Any images you choose are right. It's your vision and anything goes

- If you get stuck, think about things you don't want and find words and images that represent the opposite! For example:

YOU DON'T WANT THIS	THE OPPOSITE IMAGE MIGHT BE THIS
Low energy	✓ A woman jogging or playing a sport
To feel heavy, burdened	✓ A woman leaping (find a tampon ad) :)
To feel moody	✓ A woman smiling authentically
Stress	✓ A beach
"This is gonna be hard!"	✓ A finish line
Fat thighs	✓ Skinny jeans!

It's time to take a deep breath, because you've reached another milestone. Time to sign off for an hour, a day, a week, or more and start creating your vision board. Really take your time to make this special and beautiful, and remember, think big!

After your work of art is done, make sure it's utilized properly. Mount your board in a place where you'll see it several times a day. This can be in your bedroom, office, kitchen, even your bathroom! If it's virtual, maybe use it as your desktop picture, or on your phone or tablet so you can refer to it easily. You can make it private or accessible to others, but wherever you decide it will be, ensure that it's a spot you see often.

My board is mounted to a wall in my bedroom. Each morning I have a couple deep breaths in front of it to center myself. I also have a picture of it on my mobile phone and it's my laptop screen saver. I have a note that summarizes my vision in my wallet. This might seem a little much from your perspective, but from my angle, I'm doing what I need to keep connected to what's important to me. As shared in chapter one (b), self-accountability has a better chance when you are connected to the goal emotionally. My vision board helps me anchor that.

Remember! The purpose of the vision board is to constantly remind you of your dreams and goals.

Chapter 2: Keys to G

- Picturing what you want is key to getting it. The more clearly you create a clear goal within you, the easier it is to reach for it. Make this happen for yourself. Only you can.

- Follow through! You have now both written your vision and created it in pictures.

- Know your vision board upside down and backwards. Memorize the words and feel the emotion that you felt when you made it, whether you feel proud, strong, energetic, resourceful, brave, etc. Study your board numerous times a day. And own it in your soul.

3

SHOPPING FOR LINGERIE

Yay! It's my turn to talk! I'm Michelle, your tell-it-like-it-is-super-fantastic-nutritionist! Let's dive right in.

As a business owner, I'm constantly scanning publications hoping to spark cool new ideas about how to grow my business. I recently happened upon an article called "14 Things Every Successful Person Has In Common" and I started thinking about my most successful clients. What traits or characteristics do they share?

Sure, that article was written with a business focus, but qualities can apply to any goal reached. It makes no difference if you're trying to make money on the stock market, start your own business or lose weight—the concepts are the same.

Here are some of those traits:

- Successful people set goals to allow them clarity for what's required to accomplish them.

- They're more excited about the journey than the payout.

- They take accountability for themselves and their actions.

So, here's my approach to set you up for success using these exact same principles!

Trait #1: Setting Goals That CAN Be Accomplished

How do you plan to get to the finish line if you don't know where the finish line is? You can't!

It's like saying you're going to run a race but have no idea where it begins and ends, let alone the length of the route. People who are successful have a plan, a map, a blueprint… something to guide them on their journey, whatever journey that might be. You picked up this book because you want to accomplish something; maybe it's losing 5, 10 or 50 pounds, perhaps it's getting a better understanding of your emotional ties to food.

Or maybe you don't even know what the goal is; you just know you want to make a change.

Either way, it's time to formulate a plan and set some S.M.A.R.T. goals!

First, if you have your own method of creating a plan that works, by all means, stick with it. If you think you have your own method of creating a plan that works, but if you're reading this and it's not working, you obviously haven't come up with the right method! Let me help.

When working with clients, we always ensure our action plan is clearly outlined. The system we've found works best and is easy to remember is S.M.A.R.T., which, in business speak, stands for Specific, Measurable, Actionable, Realistic and Timely.

Another approach—and this one makes me smile—suggests S.M.A.R.T stands for Specific, Measurable, Accountable, Resonant and Thrilling. Hey, it's your plan, so use whatever acronym works for you!

Here's an example of what your S.M.A.R.T. goal template can look like, including the definition of each category:

	SPECIFIC DESIRED OUTCOME (AKA GOAL)	MEASURABLE	ACTIONS ACCOUNTABLE	REALISTIC (RESONANT)	TIMING (THRILLING)
D E F I N I T I O N	In this area capture the goal you want to develop/accomplish.	List the "how" you'll know this has been achieved; for example, evaluation, testing, exhibiting, presenting skills, mastery, etc.	List what needs to be done to get you to your end goal here.	Update progress on goal here. If this doesn't reflect what was listed for the last two columns, adjust your plan to what's realistic.	Identify a timeline for each step.
S A M P L E	Purchase my first car within six months.	1. Save $500/ month for a deposit 2. Put together payment plan with down payment in mind and stick to this	1. Get insurance quotes (ensure you qualify) 2. Decide on make/model (other details) 3. Decide on leasing or financing options (and get approved) 4. Ensure monthly payments can be met by making a monthly budget (gas, insurance, car payments)		Month 1: 1. Get insurance quote 2. Decide on make/model and price out car 3. Design budget to meet monthly savings Month 7: 4. Ensure $3000 saved, order car 5. Stick to monthly budget of X to ensure car payments can be made

Let's say I wanted to buy my first car. I could say to you, "Hey, I'm gonna save up to buy a car," and you might say "Wow! That's so cool—but how do you plan to do it?" Hmmmm…. good point.

Applying the S.M.A.R.T. plan system, you'd say instead: "Hey, I'm gonna save up to buy a car. To do this, I will save $500 a month for six months in order to put a $3000 deposit on a Toyota Camry."

Clearly, the second statement is more realistic, specific and concrete.

The same opportunity applies for you to create your own personal S.M.A.R.T. system for your own health goals.

Here's a sample of a plan directed towards dropping some of that irritating, running-too-much-of-my-life body fat. Feel free to use some of these ideas, or design something unique to yourself. Note that I've included a spot for you to record your reward for reaching your goal.

	SPECIFIC DESIRED OUTCOME (AKA GOAL)	MEASURABLE	ACTIONS (ACCOUNTABLE)	REALISTIC (RESONANT)	TIMING (THRILLING)
S A M P L E	20 lbs lost in 90 days (Insert target date here) _____	a) Step on scale once per week to ensure I'm on track for my end of week goal b) Send my nutritionist (Michelle) a weekly food log for feedback c) Get body composition testing done at local facility	a) Monday, Wednesday a.m. boot camp, Saturday morning spin class b) Total avoidance of alcohol and chocolate for 30 days, 2 treats per week thereafter c) Send food log weekly to Michelle and Nancy	a) Meal plan once per week b) Grocery shop once per week c) Meal prep twice per week with groceries (Sunday and Wednesday) d) Gym 3x/ week for 45 min and yoga 1x/week	a) 10 lbs down in 30 days (2.5 lbs per week) Reward: _____ b) 20 lbs down in 60 days (approx. 1.25 lbs/week) Reward: _____
	Lose 2.5 lbs per week in first 30 days and 1.25 lbs thereafter per week	Step on scale once per week to ensure loss	a) E-mail BFF (or Michelle) with food log and weekly weight for accountability	a) Sugar-free for week one to get rid of cravings; 2 treats per week thereafter b) See above actions c) Make sure I eat dinner no later than 7:30 p.m. and no snacks after 4) Drink 8 cups of water and 1 green tea per day	a) Stand in front of mirror in bra and panties (with my hair and makeup done). Note 8 changes that make me feel great (things that are different or better) Reward: what this feels like! Stay here until what I see connects with me inside. Feel the, "I've got this!" and carry that feeling with me.

Remember, each person is blessed with their own set of strengths and weaknesses (and yes, I did say blessed; a weakness is often a blessing in disguise), so only you can really map out your goal and how you plan to achieve it.

Take your time. This can be a daunting task and it might take you up to a week (or more) to complete it. The beauty of this book is that you don't have to race through it to finally get started losing weight (or whatever else your healthy goal might be). Just simply moving through these steps authentically—and I mean really taking these ideas into consideration—is already getting you started on your path to success.

You go, girl!

Using the car purchase example again, think about it this way. In order to be able to buy or lease that car, you'll imagine how prepared you'll need to be before you make this big investment. You'll picture yourself making the monthly payments on time and taking on the extra responsibility of owning a car.

You'll also do some due diligence before making the leap. If this is your first car, you might seek guidance from a professional or a friend or family member on the technicalities of making a major purchase like this. They, in turn, would most likely recommend getting quotes for car payments and insurance. Building a budget that factors in these costs as well as gas expenses would allow you to understand what you need to have saved monthly in order to feasibly own this car.

My point is (I promise I'll get there!) is that often, actions need to be taken ahead of time to set you up for success. In the case of losing weight, the steps outlined in this book are meant to prepare your brain to think about important issues like your emotional connections to food and re-evaluate your typical thinking on matters related to health and your body. If you put the time in now to think about this, your path to success will be a lot less rocky. Pinky swear!

Now it's your turn to get S.M.A.R.T. (but for now, hold off filling out what you think your reward might be, we will get to that).

You can find this exercise in the workbook!

=>> http://bonus.weightlossgspot.com

	SPECIFIC DESIRED OUTCOME (AKA GOAL)	MEASURABLE	ACTIONS (ACCOUNTABLE)	REALISTIC (RESONANT)	TIMING (THRILLING)
S A M P L E	Limit treats to 2 per week	a) Track treats on food log	a) Highlight treats consumed so they stand out on the food log b) If for whatever reason I have more than 2 treats, I commit to 1 extra workout per treat consumed	a) Ensure I look at social calendar at beginning of week to ensure I plan alcohol and treats accordingly	a) Use a star in my calendar for every day I'm treat-free. Watch my daily success (the star reinforcement is very much like crossing out on a task list daily). b) Count my star success any time

Congratulations! Now you have a custom plan! Doesn't that feel good?

I always tell my clients that having your plan is half the battle; you now know where you are going, how you will get there and when you should arrive. The beauty of it all is that you're in charge, so if you need to adjust your plan based on faster or slower progress, that's fine. Know that this is YOUR journey and no one else's! Get comfortable with the pace you've set for yourself.

Trait #2: Being Responsible And Accountable, Today And Tomorrow

"To thine own self be true."

~ Hamlet

We agree with Hamlet! But here's a question for you: when was the last time you celebrated a success or owned up to a failure?

When we have kids, we celebrate every single one of their milestones: the first step, the first word, the first day of school, the first hockey goal.

What I want to know is this—why does this recognition have to end? When we get to a certain age, not only do we stop celebrating, we often skip even acknowledging our achievements. Imagine how much different a win, YOUR win, would feel if you acknowledged it by sharing it with someone else and taking the moment you deserve to soak it in with an, "I did it! I worked my tail off on this and not only did I pull it off, I did it well! Yahoo to me! I rule!"

Make a note of this: LEARN to celebrate YOU. On second thought, just making note of it isn't enough. You need a plan! Let's make a list of what celebrating how awesome you are would look like. Do it right now.

Nancy here: I have a couple of ideas to get you started.

- *Call a friend and tell them of your success. Be specific. Tell them what you did that was terrific and WOWie for you!*

- *Grab your journal. Write about your pride. Record things like what it feels like in the moment. How did you do this for yourself? What makes you worth it? And what would more of this success do for your life?*

- *Go for a walk. Breathe in the fresh air. Enjoy and consider every step. Enjoy and consider you, your effort, your success, your new way of BEing.*

These are three ways I acknowledge my successes. For me, a fourth would be sharing that milestone with my boys. It's important to me to teach them the importance of self-recognition, too!

Your turn, now, to come up with celebration ideas of your own (make sure you write this down in the workbook)!

_____

_____

_____

This is all great. But hold up for a second. What if (gasp) we're not successful?

Instead of wallowing, why not use this as another tool in our journey? Too often, we neglect to acknowledge why a plan didn't pan out like we thought it would.

You could also choose to simply ignore your unreached goal—but we bet you'll never forget.

Other easy coping mechanisms include blaming others, outside conditions or just plain bad luck for lack of success.

Here's the truth: you and you alone hold the key to both your successes and your failures.

Outside influences might distract you, slow you down or give you new perspective, but you ultimately choose whether or not you're defeated.

Deciding to take responsibility and accountability for every thought and action is liberating. Scary, for sure, but liberating! Whether you announce this to the world or just in your private thoughts, taking accountability of your own stuff means you also get to choose your own stuff.

So, for the purposes of this book, since we already know all about our stuff from authentically completing the exercises in Chapters 1 and 2, let's move on and make sure you're ready to take responsibility and accountability for everything on this journey.

Let's measure your determination!

You Know You Want It

You're here for a reason. Time for you to own it!

Own it in your soul. I LOVE this saying. LOVE IT. No more of this so-so, vanilla-flavoured living. You bought this book for a reason. My guess is that your Here has haunted you most of your adult life. But guess who's to blame for the haunting? Yep, that would be you, my friend.

It's the moment of truth. You need to choose right now. Are you gonna stay or go? Play or pass? Participate and enjoy the ride of your life or keep watching the life you want from the bleachers? You are the only one who has the power to do this!

Now's the time to decide if you want to commit 100% by taking accountability for all your actions. Otherwise, you may as well close this book!

And remember, 100% means you will follow through with actions and take responsibility for doing so. As Jack Canfield says in his book, The Success Principles, "99% is a Bitch and 100% is a Breeze."

Phew! You're still here? That is awesome! I'm so glad. Welcome to the rest of your life. And welcome to discovering YOUR Weight Loss G-Spot!

Your task now is to fold this page down. Read it every morning until you believe it. Read it every night until you automatically recite it like a bedtime prayer.

Okay, enough with the deep thoughts and the reading and the exploring, for now. It's time for some action, both in the bedroom and in this weight loss process!

You'll find here a list of actions that are key for you to get from Here to your finish line.

Some you'll do once and some you'll commit to doing weekly, but I promise the combination will get you from Point A (today) to Point G— the G-Spot of weight loss.

Actions include:

- Weekly weigh-ins

- Measuring your hip-to-waist ratio

- A visual reminder of you're Here (yes this means it's picture time)

- Completing your Weekly Wellness Tracker

- Completing Your G-Spot Symptoms Checker before and after your weight loss journey

You can download the Weekly Wellness Tracker and the G-Spot Symptom checker here:

http://bonus.weightlossgspot.com/

You'll also need to:

Buy a reliable digital scale. This will give you an idea of how your weight is changing week to week. Pick one day of the week (the best day based on your own schedule) and at the same time each week (before food or drink), step on that scale and record on your Weekly Wellness Tracker.

> *Nancy here: Did you register that request? Michelle said weigh yourself ONCE a week and once only. Choose your time and your day. Weighing yourself daily is INSANE. Weighing yourself multiple times a day is an illness. Be fair to yourself. Be real with yourself. Manage yourself. I repeat, weigh yourself once a week only!*

Take another deep, cleansing breath here. For many people (Nancy included), the weigh-in can be a time of panic, self-loathing or downright disgust. Please don't do this to yourself!

The point here is just to set a baseline—not to confirm whether you are 10, 20 or 50 pounds above where you think you should be. Record this number in the space indicated on the Symptoms Checker.

Please do this one morning at your convenience before you have consumed any food or drink. Record it below as well.

Date: _____

Weight: _____

Remember, this is just a starting place. This is a temporary number and you are on a path to reduce this and get healthy!

> *Nancy here. I haven't had a scale in my home for over 20 years. Like I'm not hard enough on myself as it is when I get up in the morning and look in the mirror! Why add to that with a scale? To fulfill Michelle's request, I weigh-in at a friend's house. She keeps me honest. Remember, we need to know where we are, to know how to get where we want to go. Another reminder: do this ONCE A WEEK only!*

Bio Impedance Analysis: If you are inspired to collect more baseline data for yourself, consider getting a Bio Impedance Analysis (BIA). This machine measures body fat, muscle mass, hydration, as well as a host of other health indicators.

Often health clubs, chiropractors, naturopaths and even some medical doctors carry these machines and can run the test for a nominal fee.

This is one of the most accurate ways to measure fat loss and is a great adjunct to the scale and measuring tape.

If you live in Oakville, Ontario (and surrounding areas) and would like this test, please accept a complimentary test at my clinic. Please contact michelle@strongnutritionandweightloss.com

As mentioned above, fill out the G-Spot Symptom Checker. This handy-dandy questionnaire will allow you to hone in on any other physical stuff that may be dragging you down.

Fill this out twice: today and then after you've lost the weight. Compare the two questionnaires and look at how different they are once a healthy lifestyle becomes a priority in your life!

Tip: Consider the fact that muscle weighs more than fat. If you gain muscle and lose an equal amount of fat, you will not see this weight loss reflected on the scale; in fact you might even see a slight increase on the scale. A scale is a valuable tool to allow you to track progress, but knowing your hip to waist ratio helps provide a really reliable measurement of weight loss and body composition.

Take Hip And Waist Measurements

A flexible tape measure is the second accountability tool you'll need. Measuring your hip and waist areas allows you to determine if you carry more fat around your mid-section than around your hips and thighs.

Of course, you can tell if this is the case by looking in the mirror, but measuring is always helpful so you can tell if these inches are going down over time. Carrying fat around your belly is one significant indicator of your predisposition to chronic disease, like stroke and heart attack. So the goal is to decrease your overall fat content in your body, but specifically from around your belly.

How the heck do I measure my hips and waist, you ask?

1. Measure, using the flexible tape, at the narrowest part of your waist, or right above your belly button. Write this number down on your G-Spot Symptoms Checker.

2. Next, stand with your feet together and measure at the widest part of your hips, making sure to capture your buttocks. Write this number in the space indicated on the G-Spot Symptoms Checker. If you haven't done so already, you can download the G-Spot Symptom Checker here: http://bonus.weightlossgspot.com/

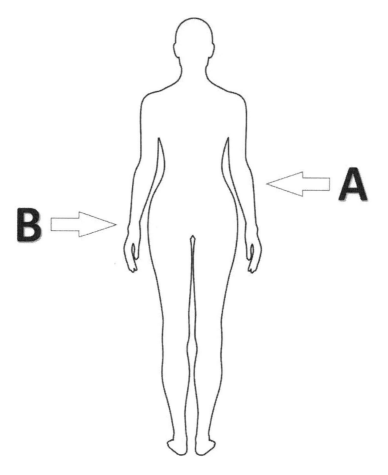

Now fill in the blanks: A ____ / B____= _____ your waist-to-hip ratio.

For example, say your waist measures 36 inches and your hips measure 45 inches.

Divide 36 by 45 and you get 0.8. Your waist-to-hip ratio is 0.8.

Fact: New promising research shows that women with a waist of equal to or greater than 88cm (35 inches) or a ratio of 0.8 or higher have a greater risk of developing cardio-metabolic conditions like heart diseases, than women with a smaller waist-to-hip ratio. By the way, having a heart attack or a stroke definitely isn't sexy.

Prove Your Progress

Usually we try to hide photographic evidence of our extra weight, but for this journey, it's important to be able to see where you have come from, so having proof is key. A picture is worth a thousand words; it allows you to go back and see how far you have come. You can even use it as a motivational tool (who was that chick in the picture?) to remind yourself where you won't ever go again. What you do with your picture and how you reference it is up to you.

Here are a couple of ideas: If the picture is digital, make a "G-Spot" file on your computer to store relevant data from this journey. If you decide to print your pic, put it somewhere you can see it on a daily basis.

Either way, know that when this book is done and your journey is complete, you'll be looking at someone new, someone who has changed, mind and body.

Track It!

Keeping a record is key to hitting Your Weight Loss G-Spot. You've got to be clear on the path that got you successfully to your goal so you can go back again and again and again.

Not only does this hold you accountable to yourself, but can also hold you accountable to us, or to a friend or family member. How would your decisions change if you knew you had to report to someone else? Whether you police yourself or we do it as a team, daily recordings of your food, drink, exercise and sleep is extremely important to keeping you mindful of your actions.

It is my firm belief that tracking foods yields higher success rates of fat loss. Studies confirm this, like the one done at Kaiser Permanente's Center for Health Research in Portland, Oregon. Lead author Jack Hollis, Ph.D., reports that during the weight loss process, "the more food records people kept, the more weight they lost and those who kept daily food records lost twice as much weight as those who kept no records."

Nancy here: I am so not a fan of the word hate, but here's the truth—I HATE tracking my food. Hate it. It's like a slap in the face. It haunts me. It drives me crazy. It makes me feel bad. It confirms my greatest fear that I suck. Is this sounding familiar? Then go reread the page I told you to fold down. Read it as many times as you need to, until you get it that this is no longer a choice. This is the price of participation. It's the key to the ignition of the car. Please continue, Michelle.

Thank you, Nancy. And now, here are some suggestions about how to track your food.

Whatever method you prefer to track your food is fine, as long as it works for you. Use scrap paper, or the notes app into your smart phone, my fitness pal is a popular app you could use or print off our Weekly Wellness Tracker.

If you want some accountability, submit your food log to me as part of your personal support system!

Do You Need A Push? We Are Here To Help!

Option #1 Food-Based Accountability

If you are someone who needs that extra little bit of support and accountability in the food department, this is for you!

What you get:

Individualized support from me, Michelle, your nutritionist!

Weekly accountability to help you achieve Your Weight Loss G-Spot

A personalized review of food logs, plus comments for improvements

Peace of mind, knowing that you're making awesome decisions!

Want to know more? Contact Michelle at michelle@strongnutritionandweightloss.com

Option #2 Own It In My Soul Accountability

If you've been nodding your head in recognition and agreement throughout this book so far, but haven't started your journey yet, it's time for some coaching that will kick start your head and your heart into action!

What you get:

Six individual coaching sessions from me, Nancy, your Connection Coach

Daily accountability check-ins (as needed)

This book's content, customized to your individual needs through coaching

The support of someone who gets it, with the ability to help you overcome self-created hurdles

Want to know more? Contact Nancy at Nancy@nancymilton.ca

However you decide to track your food, you MUST fill out your form whenever you eat and drink! Don't wait until the end of your long day. Instead, take breaks and record it over the course of the day. Filling it out at the end of each day is cheating. And we all know cheating sucks! You've done that enough in the health department. You're way better than that, girlfriend.

Nancy here: Personally, recording my food and drink intake helps push me to make better food choices. Hence me not liking to record it!

Trait #3: Getting Excited About The Journey

Now that we know what the finish line looks like, let's make sure we're ready to start.

It's easy to say, "I'm starting Monday," or "I'm gonna lose 20 pounds," but what will make you STICK to this goal? Saying it is easy, but living it day in and day out can be hard.

Everyone's gung ho in the first two weeks. Then real life sets in and these changes can feel mundane and annoying. I get it. I watch many clients go through this. Here's my advice: accept and make peace with the fact that weight loss isn't instantaneous (but it's doable—see box).

Note: When it comes to weight loss, it's possible that your weight may stay the same or even go up for no real notable reason from week to week. Know that there are many variables that can affect weight loss, including hormones, stress, sleep, exercise; weight loss is not simply just about calories in versus calories out. Typically, people lose about 1 to 3 lbs per week when following our guide. This could be less or more on any given week; the goal is that weight is going down in general over time.

Keep It Interesting Along The Way!

Enjoy the process because in essence, every step is one closer to getting to your finish line. If you aren't in love with the journey, how can you expect to maintain it once you've arrived? The journey is half the battle (if not more). Plus, the journey forms the habits that will keep you on track in the future.

Nancy here: I'll share yet another personal story with you.

I used to be a wimp when it came to long car rides. Picture a dog panting at the window wanting to be let outside. That's what I was like. Imagine how much fun I'd be to travel with. To keep from going insane, I had to switch it up for me and for the people in the car with me.

Now, before I leave, I research potential spots to stop so we always have options for short reprieves. I have snacks I look forward to, games I can play in the car like Table Talker, things I can do with my hands like knitting, quilting, even cleaning out my purse!

The bottom line: not only am I good to travel by car now, I organize the trips myself!

The message is this: the journey is yours. Make it what you want it to be!

And here's a personal story from me:

For my nutrition practice, one of my big goals was to be on TV to teach people about health and nutrition. I wanted to inspire wellness on a grand scale. In order to get there, I knew that I needed to be an expert in my field. Part of developing those skills involved working one-on-one with clients to give me exposure to many different health issues. This also helped me learn to communicate differently based on unique personalities and kept me very connected to the industry.

I love meeting new people and love coaching clients through whatever health goal they have. I've realized that you really have to love the process, because chances are it's going to take some time to get to your goal. In addition to seeing clients, I have small and large projects on the go (this book, for example) that further my learning, open new doors and give me skills I wouldn't have had if I hadn't taken on these tasks. Part of our journey is getting excited about all the little things you're going to do along the way to set yourself up for success.

An update: just so you know, I've since been blessed with many opportunities to speak on TV about my passion for health and wellness. So I'm getting there and you will too!

When things get hard and you're thinking about packing it in, you need to think about what you'll tell yourself or what you'll do to get re-motivated? Capture 10 things below or in your workbook that you will do to get excited (or re-excited) about your journey:

_____

_____

_____

Success Indicators

Trust me when I say this: you need to have a goal and a plan for the road ahead. It will get bumpy, there might be roadblocks and sometimes you might even want to turn off the ignition and shut right down.

Every one of us is different in how we judge our success. If it's weight loss you're after, indicators are as simple as whether you've reached your weight loss goal for the period of time you've set. For other people, indicators are a measurement on a scale of 1 to 10. I ask clients to rate their symptom (e.g. whatever they want to change) on a scale. If they started at a 2/10 (where 10 is the best) and indicated they would be content at an 8/10 and with proper nutrition, fitness, sleep etc. reach this, than this is how they have measured their success.

Indicators are personal. However you decide to measure success is fine; just make sure you set your indicators ahead of time.

Another personal aside about indicators - I'm about to let you in on a secret about me. A few years into my practice, I questioned changing career paths.

It was hard. Money wasn't steady and I didn't have health benefits. I was spending a lot of money and expending a lot of energy but earning little in return. It was time for a serious reality check. I had to look deep inside and ask myself if this career was truly for me. The answer was without a doubt YES, definitely! Okay. Phew.

With that established, I knew I had to readjust my expectations of what success looked like for me. Was I after more time, more money, more recognition?

At the time, I defined success financially because I was saving to buy my first home. I knew I'd need markers of that success and small rewards along the way to keep my motivation levels up. I had an end goal: in five years, I wanted to be earning a certain amount of money annually. I disciplined myself to set both yearly and monthly markers and weekly client targets to ensure I was moving towards that ultimate goal. As long as, when each year ended, I was closer to reaching my ultimate goal, I was a happy camper. And if I wasn't on the path to reaching the goal, I knew I had to re-examine what had to be done to get me to that annual milestone.

When it wasn't quite there, I decided I needed to take on more speaking engagements. I needed to connect more on social media sites. I needed to hand out more door-to-door flyers. I needed to meet more professionals around my area to develop more referral networks. It became a game—what effort netted me the most return?

Now It's Your Turn!

If you look closely, you will see that your health goals are not so different than my goal to start and build a private nutritional coaching business.

You know you want to (insert main goal here) and you have purchased this book because you are willing to make some changes. Getting started with something new is always an exciting time.

But what happens when a month into the new you, the old you emerges, cravings hit or you overindulge at a party and don't meet your weekly goal? What happens when this new and exciting time is now just real life?

Believe me when I say this: it will happen, in one form or another. I guarantee that you will at one point cringe at the thought of "being good" (which is a term many of my clients use; please help us help you remove this phrase from your vocabulary!)

So what will be your markers of success? Indicators for weight loss can be fewer pounds on the scale, inches lost or fitting into a particular size of pants. Markers can be anything that inspires you to exclaim, "Hurray! First milestone reached!"

You got here, now it's time to celebrate.

But how?

Keep Your Eye On The Prize

Rewards. We all love them. For many, they are the driving force behind many goals met and obstacles overcome. People all over the globe, from all walks of life, live for rewards. We're offered rewards to stay loyal to certain gas companies. Other businesses offer incentives and rewards to their employees for monthly and yearly targets met and banks offer spending rewards that can be redeemed for items or discounted airfare. We all love rewards. I love them, and they work. This is why it's important to celebrate your milestones with rewards in this life-changing process.

Go back to your S.M.A.R.T. plan at the beginning of this chapter and look at your timeline section (far right of your template).

In the example given, the first milestone is 10 lb. in 30 days. You have two options here: a) you can work towards this goal, meet it, give yourself a pat on the back and move on to the next phase, or b) CELEBRATE! 10 lb. removed, feeling confident and beautiful with something super fantastic! I'd choose the second option if I were you.

But let's be clear. When we talk about rewards for goals met, let me be very specific here. I do not mean a food reward!

> *Nancy here: Michelle, did you read my mind? My reward would have totally been a large peanut butter and chocolate ice cream. And then, because my day was shot anyway, I'd stop and pick up a bakery cookie. Whoever used food as a reward when we were little was so wrong. And my guess is they didn't know any better. It's important we know what a real reward is. Listen carefully to how Michelle explains it. You need to unwind the habit of food reward and introduce rewards that really matter!*

Here are some reward ideas my clients have used:

- Give yourself a home facial or go get one!

- Get a massage (love these!)

- Take a day off work (no housework allowed!)

- Lounge alone or with your best friend bestie (or sexy man friend)

- Buy a size smaller of _____ that you now fit into.

- Journal about your success! Acknowledge it!

- Make time to book a visit with a friend

- Go for a walk somewhere peaceful

- Read a new book (I hear Fifty Shades of Grey is a sure-fire way to get closer to your G-Spot)

- Take a yoga class

- Watch some smutty, indulgent television

- Try a new recipe

- Take a picture of the evolving you and revel in the changes

- Rent a movie

- Visit an art gallery (or somewhere you love, sans children)

- Spend the day in bed sleeping, reading, being cozy

- Window shop or actually shop (this would be my treat)

- Volunteer your time for a good cause

Whatever the reward is, it needs to mean something to you. Pick something small or large, expensive or inexpensive, short-term or long; but pick something that will help motivate you to reach that next milestone within the timeline you have already set. Back you go to your S.M.A.R.T plan and fill in the blank with your reward or incentive for each of your timelines or milestones reached.

Okay, we're getting there!

Often, we jump into new projects with gusto and don't bother to take the time to set ourselves up properly for success. Knowing your baseline, where you started from, where you are going and making sure you are prepared for the journey is just as important as getting to your finish line. Consider the fact that getting there might be more arduous without having put in the due diligence!

Up until now, we've been setting you up for success. I would argue getting to this point is a success in itself, so way to go! Let's keep going! Remember this is all building you up to help you get to Your Weight Loss G-Spot.

Before moving forward, make sure you've taken these steps:

- Download a blank S.M.A.R.T. goals template from the link bellow.

- Download the Weekly Wellness Tracker and start using it.

- Take a before picture of yourself and keep it somewhere handy.

- Measure and calculate your waist to hip ratio.

- Buy a scale and use it. *Nancy here: with a vow to use it WEEKLY only!*

- Complete your vision board and reference it daily.

- Weigh yourself weekly and capture the measurement on your Weekly Wellness Tracker.

- Fill in your G-Spot Symptoms Checker before and after your weight loss journey through this book.

All resources can be downloaded here:

http://bonus.weightlossgspot.com/

Chapter 3: Keys to G

- Take the time to first understand what's prevented you from finding success so far; then you can finally release those barriers for today and your future. This release can be like a flashlight in a dark tunnel of Your Weight Loss G-Spot quest...

- Although it was work, completing the above to-do list was a HUGE leap to you getting to where you want to be. Remember, preparation is key. You have to get your head AND heart activated in this process. You deserve nothing less!

4

SEARCHING FOR — AND FINDING — THE MAGIC

Michelle here again… Are you ready to see your kitchen through the eyes of a nutritionist?

"By failing to prepare, you are preparing to fail."

~Benjamin Franklin

For many of us, the kitchen represents a dangerous place. Temptation lurks at every turn. We know we can choose to create awesome, healthy meals but we don't know how to start. We might even view our kitchen as a daunting space, a foreign, unknown land of herbs, spices, gadgets and gizmos.

What if, instead, our kitchen was a place that represented simplicity, comfort and health? A place where we create great food with ease; a place that represents all the good things in life—socializing with friends and family, vitality, peace and of course, health.

Here's the good news. Your kitchen can be all of this and more… if you let us help you get there!

You just need to trust me. Are you on board?

65

Good. Because before we go any further, we need to cover some groundwork that will allow you to understand the definition of whole, real foods. Knowing the basics will allow you to make more informed decisions when you're faced with the confusing world of grocery shopping. Since we're working towards a really specific goal of weight loss, knowing the essentials of nutrition will help you sort out what belongs and what doesn't fit in your personal health-promoting, fat-dropping, spirit-feeding, awesomeness-inspiring new way of living!

The **ABCD's** of Nutrition: Your Roadmap for Chapter 4

A is for Awareness:

- Cocky carbs

- Fabu fats

- Powerful proteins

B is for Bag It:

- De-mystifying labels

- Bag it and boot it

C is for Consume It:

- Master "eat-this" list

- Specific product recommendations (protein powder and bars)

- Your condiment solution

D is for Drink It:

- Your unofficial fourth macronutrient

A Is For Awareness

Here's a question: how often are you actually mindful of the choices you make? How many times in a day do you stop and really take stock of what you're doing?

More often than not, we run on robot-like autopilot, habitually going about our days with little to no consciousness about what's really happening.

Consider your morning shower for example (and hey, what an opportunity to explore your G!). When was the last time you were actually aware of how the hot water feels pouring over your body, how your scalp responds when you scrub it, how refreshed you are when you get out and towel off, ready to face the day?

The absence of mindfulness is autopilot, and autopilot will not get you to your weight loss G-Spot. In fact, autopilot in bed is what Nancy calls bread and butter sex. Vanilla sex? Ugh and ew!

Being aware or mindful of what we're doing puts a whole new spin on day-to-day activities and forces us to contemplate what would otherwise be mindless decisions.

Wake up to this idea: Before you can change your lifestyle, your weight, or whatever it is you're going for, you need to be aware of what the heck you're doing in the first place. DUH!

I would argue that one of the first steps of awareness is education. Unless you understand the basics behind any concept, the chances of you buying into it and following through are slim to none.

In my practice, I spend a lot of time educating my clients. I share with clients WHAT the answer is and WHY I recommend it. This education enables you to make better and more informed decisions when you're on your own.

Let's apply this concept to your kitchen. Instead of being tormented by it, own it! Be the boss of your kitchen! Even though it seems hard, take the steps to learn what you need to do and why you need to do it; and start with the fundamentals (a.k.a. nutrition!).

Here's the scientific stuff that will arm you with all the ammunition you'll need to understand food, and then apply your knowledge to make awesome choices.

Ready to dive in? Let's do this!

First, let's go over the basics.

All foods are made up of a mixture of three macronutrient groups: fats, proteins and carbohydrates. Some foods have more of one group than another. For example, chicken is made up predominately of protein, but also contains some fats.

For you to really hit your G-Spot in the kitchen you need to be cool with all three of these groups.

Let's talk carbs.

Carbohydrates, a.k.a. Cocky Carbs

Carbs have earned a bad rap (and for good reason in many cases) and many of us cringe at the thought of enjoying them, thinking we'll gain weight instantly.

But what do you consider a carb? We tend to associate them with processed foods like breads, pasta, crackers and so on. What we fail to realize is that carbs come in more forms than just white French baguettes and warm cinnamon rolls (try not to drool too much on your book pages).

Did you know? Fruits are also considered simple carbohydrates, but these natural, unprocessed fructose-based sugars do not enter the bloodstream quite as quickly. Due to the fibre content, vitamins and minerals, although technically simple in nature, fruits (in moderation) are a healthy part of a food plan.

Technically—yawn—carbohydrates are sugars. Essentially, the body uses carbohydrates in different foods to make glucose, which can be used immediately for energy or stored in your body for later use. There are two forms of carbohydrates, simple and complex, that you can get these sugars from. Where can you find them?

Have a look at a few examples.

SIMPLE CARBS	COMPLEX CARBS
White bread	Quinoa
White Potatoes	Beans and lentils
Sugary treats like pop and pastries	Yams and beets

For those of you worrying that carbs will create that dreaded expansion of the waistline, you're right to avoid white breads, white pastas, pop, candy, syrups, pastries, and so on and so on and so on.

In simple terms, here's all you need to know:

Simple carbs = your healthy body's kryptonite

Complex carbs = your go-all-night-long fuel (yeah, baby!)

Nancy here: so Michelle calls the next paragraph the boring stuff because she knows we just want to know enough to get the weight off, yes? But I want to challenge you here. Read and reread this. Empower yourself to own that it's you, YOU who does this to your body and your mind. You create the emotional rollercoaster. You want to be an expert in the kitchen? Use that counter space for finding the G? Then read this. Get this. Make you a priority.

I'm back and I know this seems dry and boring but it really does help to know how all of this stuff works. I promise. Take the time to consider all of the scientific facts, and you'll feel better about the decisions you're making.

Ready to go back to school? Here we go:

CODE WORDS FOR SUGAR

WATCH OUT FOR THESE BAD BOYS; THEY ARE DISGUISED ON MANY LABELS!

Agave
Barley malt syrup
Beet sugar
Brown rice syrup
Brown sugar cane crystals (or, even better, "cane juice crystals")
Cane sugar
Coconut sugar and coconut palm sugar
Corn sweetener
Corn syrup, or corn syrup solids
Dehydrated cane juice
Dextrin
Dextrose
Evaporated cane juice
Fructose
Fruit juice concentrate
Glucose
High-fructose corn syrup
Honey
Invert sugar
Lactose
Maltodextrin
Malt syrup
Maltose
Maple syrup
Molasses
Palm sugar
Raw sugar
Rice syrup
Sorghum or sorghum syrup
Sucrose
Stevia
Syrup
Treacle
Turbinado sugar

Chemically, carbs are made up of one or two sugars. Therefore, they're quickly digested and easily absorbed. When too much sugar enters the bloodstream too quickly, it results in overproduction of a hormone called insulin.

The main job of insulin is to keep blood sugars at a healthy level. If it is overproduced due to excessive intake of simple carbs, than too much sugar enters your cells and your blood sugar becomes low.

This results in that "Yuck, when can I go home?" 2 to 4 p.m. slump we all know and hate. It's the result of sugars dropping too low. This plunge can push us to reach for something with caffeine or sugar (simple carbs) to curb our fatigue, our irritability, our headache and our general lousy feeling. You get what I'm throwing down here?

The following diagram represents a general depiction of what happens to your body when you eat a few too many simple carbs.

You decide you're going to indulge in just one decadent chocolate chip cookie after lunch. Follow what happens here:

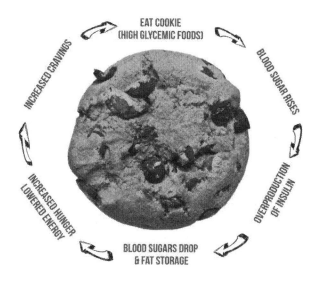

YUM! Sugar enters blood stream quickly

Blood sugar rises

Insulin is produced

Too much blood sugar = too much insulin produced

Too much insulin = too much sugar entering cells

Results in low blood sugar and fat storage

Low blood sugar = general fatigue and cravings for simple sugars SO

You consume more simple sugars

Repeat cycle!

Recap: This "cookie plunge" is dangerous. When you eat too many simple carbs, your body is triggered to eat more. This cycle makes you overeat, creates a blood sugar and hormonal imbalance and ultimately leads to weight gain!

Listen up! The key to Your Weight Loss G-Spot is making complex carbs a larger part of your life versus just consuming the simple ones.

What will this mean for you? Less of a sugar spike, therefore less of a downward plunge, plus sustainable energy that's way better for the smarter, peppier you! Plus, let's get real – you won't want to hunt for your G-Spot if you are so tired!

What you need to know:

Simple sugars are often processed and high in refined flours and sugars. Ditch these: table sugar, fruit juices, brown sugars, white breads, pastas, crackers, alcohol (Don't panic! You can enjoy alcohol with care; we'll talk more about this later) and pastries.

Complex carbs are your new best friends! Welcome them (in moderation). They're high in fibre and provide long-lasting energy. Choose these: beets and yams, legumes, vegetables, and whole grains like quinoa and brown rice.

Fabu Fats

Why is fat such a dirty word?

We've become so programmed to avoid fat that we've forgotten what it actually is and how vital it is to our survival! At 9 calories per gram, twice the amount provided by protein or carbohydrates, fat provides us with energy so our bodies can function properly. Functions like brain development, synthesizing fat-soluble vitamins, protection or insulation of organs all depends on fat intake.

When you think about fat, what do you think about? I bet not the nourishing, anti-inflammatory benefits of fats like avocado and olive oil! Our aversion to fat, I believe, stems from our limited knowledge about this nutrient. It seems that often good and bad fats are lumped together in our vocabulary (check out the list below for examples of healthy versus unhealthy fats). It's time to change this now!

In my experience, many people have little to no idea that fat from olive oil and fat from potato chips are polar opposites; in proper amounts, olive oil is a fantastic food while chips are generally full of trans fats, processed sugars and unnecessary salts.

It's not really our fault; we've been bombarded with advertisements warning us that fat is bad and that "low fat" products will somehow make us thin. However, the reality of the situation is that low fat foods tend to have much more sugar than whole fat foods; fat adds flavour, so when it's removed, sugar is added. Excess sugar will eventually be stored as fat, thus fuelling the ongoing cycle of weight gain.

It's a never-ending battle for the majority of North Americans hoping to lose that tire ring around their midsection!

To summarize: low fat doesn't necessarily mean low sugar or even healthy, for that matter.

Here's a helpful chart:

Type of Fat	Key points	Example	Do we need this in our diet?
TRANS FATS	Man-made fat to help keep foods shelf stable	Fries, donuts, pastries	No
SATURATED FAT	Solid at room temperature	Cream, animal fats, tropical oils like coconut oil	Yes, in moderation and ideally from plant-based sources
UNSATURATED FAT	Composed of mono and poly unsaturated fats Mainly from plant sources	Avocado, nuts, flax, fish	DON'T FEAR THIS FAT!

As one of the three macronutrients, fat should be an integral part of our diet and not something to fear. In proper amounts, healthy fats like avocado keep us feeling fuller longer, reducing the urge to pick up processed foods (simple sugars) as a quick fix for hunger or fatigue.

In addition, healthy fat is also low on the glycemic index—meaning that it will not spike our blood sugar and leave us tired and irritable a few hours later (good news for your co-workers or life partners!).

What many do not realize is that the highs and lows created by consuming simple sugars actually makes our bodies go into starvation mode and store carbohydrates as fat.

Here's a handy chart for healthy versus unhealthy fat sources. Clip it out and bring it to the grocery store:

DITCH THESE	GRAB THESE
Margarine	Olive oil (olives)
Shortening	Avocado (and oil)
Trans fats e.g. hydrogenated oils	Flaxseed (and oil)
Lard	Raw nuts (and oils)
Fries (anything deep fried)	Raw seeds (and oils)
Donuts	Grape seed oil
Fatty cuts of meat like bacon (sorry)	Cold water fish (salmon, cod)
Ice cream (except on special occasions)	Fish oil supplements
Processed snack foods like crackers, chips, microwave popcorn	Hemp seeds

The Incredible Power Of Protein

To understand the importance of protein in our diets, let's take a trip way back to when we were cave dwellers.

Our ancestry proves that we originated as a hunter-gatherer, meat-eating species. Over time, as our evolving brains developed, we discovered that we were able to digest cultivated cereals and grains—and so began the agricultural revolution.

Before manufacturing processes were developed, we ate exactly what our bodies needed to be healthy and happy: protein, veggies, and fruit. Sadly and ironically, the Standard American Diet (SAD) that most of us follow today is extremely high in processed grains and cereals, which are tremendously difficult to digest.

The harsh reality is, our bodies are being harmed daily because of the SAD diets we consume. The "specialty" organic, hormone-free foods available at high-end organic grocery stores are exactly what our ancestors ate and therefore closer to what our bodies crave the most. We're trying to do what's best for us and get back to eating what our bodies need to live—clean, fresh, simple foods—but it's frustrating that we have to pay a premium.

It's not right and not fair to those of us who are trying to eat better. Despite this unhappy fact, there are alternatives out there. It simply highlights the importance of getting educated on what you need to buy—and one of your best friends in this journey is going to be protein.

Protein, in all its forms, is derived from an arrangement (grouping) of building blocks called amino acids. For simplicity, let's compare these amino acids to primary paint colours; red, yellow, blue. The type and concentration of a protein is simply dependent on the combination of amino acids grouped together. Different structures (proteins) are produced from a unique string of amino acids (number and combination of paint colours). For example, combining red paint and yellow paint produces orange paint, and mixing blue and yellow paint produces green paint.

Amino acids work in a similar fashion; there are just more of them, 20 in total. Of these 20 amino acids, 9 are essential, meaning you get these from foods.

The other 11 amino acids are made up in our bodies on a day-to-day basis.

Feel like you're back in Grade 9 biology? Overwhelmed? Don't be! You don't need to know these amino acids by name, but just know that grouping certain amino acids together distinguishes one protein from another. It's just a different outcome from similar materials.

Here's Nancy to break it down for you.

1. *Repeat after me: "Protein is my friend. It gives me WOWie strength (to burn calories) faster than anything else in my body."*

2. *This is key to your foundation: Protein keeps your mood and hormones in check. A month with less sugar and more protein (compared to a typical month of LOTS of sugar and a bit of protein) is the difference between happy you and really annoyed and irritable you.*

3. *Protein is like bubble wrap between me and my cravings. And I deserve bubble wrap.*

4. *When in doubt, go for protein. It makes you last longer (get your head out of the gutter) - by this, I mean it gives you long lasting energy.*

That's my Coles Notes version of protein. Now, back to Michelle to give you the technical side.

Why Protein Is A Must-Have For Finding Your Weight Loss G-Spot

Protein helps build metabolically active tissue (a.k.a. muscle). And the more muscle you have, the more calories you burn at rest. How handy is that! The truth is, we women are not programmed to bulk up, so stop worrying that you'll look like Arnold. Do yourself a favour and start increasing your servings of lean, clean protein.

Here Are Five Proteins That Block Your G-Spot:

PROTEINS TO AVOID AT ALL COSTS	WHY MICHELLE SAYS, "DON'T GIVE IN!"	YOUR BEST ALTERNATIVE IF THIS BREAKS YOUR HEART
BACON	High in preservatives, sodium and super-duper fatty!	✓ Organic bacon or even better, organic chicken or turkey bacon
SAUSAGES	Unless you know the origin of sausage meats, they are typically loaded with super gross filler ingredients and poor cuts of meat	✓ Find a butcher you trust, ask questions about raw materials and consume only occasionally
DELI MEATS	High in nasty preservatives and fillers like gluten	✓ Nitrate and nitrite-free deli meats or bake your own chicken, turkey etc. and slice the meat yourself
STORE-BOUGHT BURGERS	Generally not made with quality, lean cuts of meat	✓ Make your own in bulk and freeze. Mine are tastier anyway!
HOT DOGS	*this is just here in case you actually consider hot dogs as a meat source—they are definitely on the DENIED list!	

Protein helps to balance your blood sugars. Without it, there will be more of those afternoon slumps in energy and irritability, headaches and restless nights. Remember there are only two things you ought to be doing in bed and poor sleep isn't one of them!

Protein plays a major role in hormone synthesis. Sounds complicated, but this process is responsible for helping to build the complex network of hormones that are responsible for sleep, moods, fat burn, cravings, muscle loss or gain, concentration and so much more! Consider this: if you don't get enough protein and that results in poor sleep, how can you expect to have enough energy to make healthy choices and get active in order to lose fat?

It's all connected.

Protein keeps you feeling full and it keeps nasty cravings at bay. Compared to carbohydrates, proteins take longer to digest and therefore keep you feeling more full and satisfied. The results include less unnecessary snacking and ultimately, a reduction of overall calories. Hormonally, the satiety derived from the slower digesting proteins also keeps cravings to a minimum, which is huge for those trying to whittle away at their waistline.

Vegetarians And Vegans

I bet you thought I forgot about you!

In my clinical and private experience, I have met very few people, meat-eaters and vegan/vegetarians alike, who eat enough protein.

If you choose to live this type of lifestyle, kudos to you. Many argue that vegans and vegetarians are among the healthiest humans, presenting lower blood fat and cholesterol counts than their meat-eating counterparts. This can be true, but if you choose to live this lifestyle, just please make sure you're doing it right!

For starters, make sure you are getting enough protein. For vegetarians who eat eggs, dairy and possibly some fish, getting enough protein, once you know how much you need to have, is simple.

For all the vegans out there, you will need to get a little more creative. If you are someone who avoids all animal products, in addition to the plant-based protein options, you need to be familiar with food combining (remember the paint colour analogy?) Making sure you're knowledgeable about this will allow you to combine certain foods to create complete proteins, thus ensuring you are optimizing your diet.

Did you know? Looking back about 10,000 years ago we can see the shift from the hunter-gatherer diet that comprised mainly of meats, fresh fruits and vegetables to a diet largely dependent upon cheap, quick sources of fuel like grains and cereals. According to Paleoists, this major swing is one of the key reasons that North Americans health issues continue to increase (like heart disease and cancer) and childhood and adult obesity numbers continue to climb.

A quick visual for vegans:

Mix A + with B = P (Complete Protein)

How to combine incomplete proteins to create complete proteins

1. Combine Legumes (A) and Nuts/Seeds (B)

   eg. Kidney beans and almonds = complete protein (P)

2. Combine Grains (A) and Legumes (B)

   eg. Corn (organic preferably) and chickpeas = complete protein (P)

3. Combine Grains (A) and Nuts/Seeds (B)

   eg. Quinoa and sunflower seeds = complete protein (P)

Did you know? Almost all foods contain protein; some more than others. There are two types of proteins, incomplete and complete. Complete protein contains all the necessary amino acids necessary for optimal dietary needs, examples include eggs, fish, poultry, milk, yogurt and red meats. Incomplete protein on the other hand lack one or more of the essential amino acids, examples of incomplete protein include beans, nuts, seeds, corn, grains and peas.

At the end of the day, it doesn't matter if you choose to eat animal products or live a vegetarian or vegan lifestyle; providing the sources are clean (no junky additives like food colourings and sugar) and you eat enough of them (three main meal servings of 15-20g and 2 small snacks of 5-10g of protein), protein will forever be an amazing aid in finding Your Weight Loss G-Spot.

B Is For Bag It And Boot It

Part of getting turned on in the kitchen is ensuring that the best, most healthy foods are constantly and conveniently at your fingertips. Just as important is making sure that those processed, sabotaging foods are out of your life. If they are blocking your G-Spot, break up with them!

Demystifying Nutritional Labels

Reading the nutritional facts on any product can be a daunting task. Be your own health expert by knowing how to interpret these five essential areas on a label.

Nutrition Facts

Serving Size 1/4 Cup

Amount Per Serving

Calories 150

	% Daily Values*
Total Fat 4g	%
Saturated Fat 3g	%
Trans Fat 0g	
Total Carbohydrate	
Dietary Fiber 3g	%
Sugars 16g	

*Percent Daily Values are based on a 2,000 calorie diet.

How To Read A Nutrition Label

1. Serving size: This may be the most important factor, it is the amount considered to be one serving of the product. Pay close attention to this. The serving size can often be much smaller than what the average person might consume in one sitting. For example, the serving size for this particular food (on the label above) is ¼ cup. Let's say this label was for breakfast cereal. The reality of a person having only ¼ cup is very small. Realistically, a person could consume 1-2 cups of cereal in one sitting.

In other words, many serving sizes are arbitrary and have no basis in reality; even though a food might appear low in calories, fats and sugars, if you are having more than ¼ cup, than you will be eating upwards of two to three times the calories, fats and sugars.

The serving size represents how much of each nutrient (listed on the label) that you will get in that ¼ cup serving.

2. Calories: A calorie is a unit of energy and is different for all foods. This number represents the amount of energy we would obtain from eating the serving size of the food listed on the nutrition facts label. Calories are vital to our survival; they come from proteins, fats and carbohydrates. However, many of us are afraid of the word calorie, because our culture has taught us that consuming too many calories equals weight gain. Foods can be healthy but have high calories and other foods can be very unhealthy and be low in calories. It is the quality of the calorie that counts, plus the portion consumed!

For example, nuts and avocado are examples of high-calorie quality foods, while popsicles and diet pop are examples of low-calorie, poor quality foods.

3. Total fat: refers to the total amount of fat in the serving size, in this case it is 4g.

4. Saturated fat: refers to the total amount of saturated fat in one serving, in this case it is 3g. Saturated fats are derived from animal products and some plants like coconut, nuts and avocado. In the past we have been encouraged to avoid these fats, however, in recent years we are discovering health benefits associated with these fats. Aim to have a diet comprised of about 25% fats.

5. Trans fat: Although some fats are healthy and necessary for our diet (avocado, olive oil), others can be hazardous (trans fats). These have been linked to increased rates of heart disease. These types of fats help to extend the shelf life of products in foods like chips, pastries, fries and more; any item that contains hydrogenated oil, partially hydrogenated oil, margarine or shortening likely contains trans fats. If a package contains any of the above, the smart choice would be to avoid this.

6. Fibre: Many of us do not get enough fibre in our diet which is critical for blood sugar management, good gastrointestinal function and detoxification. Often packaged foods claim high fibre, however one would have to consume a lot of that particular food to get this high fibre, therefore checking the fibre against the serving size is key. For example, according to the label, every ¼ cup is equal to 3g of fibre. For adults, aim for a minimum of 30g of fibre per day.

Foods high in fibre include:

- beans

- lentils

- fruits and vegetables

- nuts and seeds

- whole grains like brown/wild rice, barley, oats, quinoa, bran

Did you know? Any product that contains less than 2g of fibre per serving is a product to reconsider choosing.

The way Nancy sees it- If a product has less than 2 grams of fibre per serving, skip putting it in your mouth. You'd be better off eating sand.

7. Sugar: Often we skip this and focus too much on the calorie count of a food. As we learned, a food can be healthy and high in calories at the same time. Sugar, however, is NOT a healthy product as it disrupts our immune system, causes inflammation, contributes to harmful belly fat and is devoid of any nutrients. Every 4g of sugar listed on a label is equal to 1 tsp. of sugar. So in a ¼ cup of this breakfast cereal there is about 4 tsp. of sugar. That is a lot! So if 1 cup of cereal were to be consumed, than you would be essentially eating 16 tsp. of sugar in one sitting. In my opinion, aim for as little sugar as possible through the day-less than 20g per day in my opinion.

You did it! You got through the factual nitty-gritty stuff you need to arm yourself with to take on your cravings and habits.

You now know that real foods are good, that they fuel our body and help us find our Weight Loss G-Spot. But realistically, because of our hectic schedules, some processed foods might sneak into our diets. So it's up to us to read labels carefully to keep as much junk out as possible.

Be careful here. Some nutritional facts labels can be misleading and may not paint an accurate picture of what's inside the package.

Tip: check the ingredient list for aspartame, sucralose or any other type of artificial sweetener. These man-made chemicals are calorie free and would therefore not influence the calorie count on a label. They do however stimulate cravings and the desire to eat more of that particular food than one might typically eat. Nancy here: READ THIS! Let this sink in. This is BAD. This sweetener crap screws with your body specific to cravings. Do this for yourself. Would you eat poison? Exactly.

Here's a quick story:

My girlfriend Isabelle moved to Canada from South America when she was 10. The excitement of discovering a new country and culture—let alone all the new foods to try—made every day like Christmas! She'd moved in with her sister, who quickly put parameters on the buffet of treats, which left Isa having to prioritize. Those packaged cake-like Jos Louis swiftly shot to the top of her list of favourites. At the grocery store that week, Isa begged her sister to buy the whole box of Jos Louis, after seeing ALL the other kids at school with them. Isa's sister replied, "Sure Isa! We'll buy the box as long as you can pronounce the entire ingredient list and describe what each item is."

You can guess how the story ended. Fast forward 28 years. To this day, Isa has never eaten a Jos Louis. What a great lesson her sister taught her about deciding what to put in her body!

Ingredients That Will NOT Get You To Your Weight Loss G-Spot

Beware of products that contain ingredients like MSG (monosodium glutamate), hydrogenated anything, sulphites, BHT, BHA, sodium nitrates, nitrites, food colourings (any) and acesulfame potassium. These are preservatives, additives and generally all around useless and nutritionally void of anything healthful and there are more! This is just a sampling of the goodies that lurk in our processed foods.

Tip: These 12 *"Dirty Dozen"* foods, according to the Environmental Working Group are the most highly sprayed and should be consumed organic or only after having been washed thoroughly:

Apples, strawberries, cucumber, celery, cherry tomatoes, grapes, nectarines/peaches, potatoes, spinach, bell peppers, kale/collard greens, summer squash.

Confused?

When in doubt, take a look at the label and beware:

- Ingredients ending in the letters "-ose" and "-tol" generally indicates the food is a sugar! These typically provide very few nutrients. As a general rule, be wary of ingredients like: fructose, dextrose, glucose, maltodextrin, manitol, lactose, cane sugar, cane juice, corn syrup solids, fruit juice, sorbitol, barley malt… the list goes on and on.

Here's a good rule of thumb: if you can't pronounce the name of an ingredient, chances are it is man-made!

- Look at the first few ingredients on a package. These are what the product is predominately made from. Ingredients are listed in order of their proportion within the product. If any of these ingredients are not whole foods (if you can't pronounce them), consumer beware!

Nancy's rule: if sugar is within the top FIVE ingredients on the list, put the package down!

- Steer clear of man-made sweeteners like aspartame (Equal, Nutrasweet), sucralose (Splenda), Neotame, Cyclamate (Sweet N' Low, Sugar Twin) and saccharin. They are chemicals that muck around with your hunger signals, blood sugars and energy! Last time I checked it's not sexy to fall asleep when you're getting busy.

3, 2, 1 Toss!

You're looking to make your body a sanctuary, yes? Well, the time has come to put your money where your mouth is!

Here's a step-by-step guide to transforming your kitchen into a sanctuary, which will play a direct role in you getting that much closer to reaching Your Weight Loss G-Spot (in and outside of the kitchen)!

Step 1

To prepare: Locate four large boxes. Set them on the floor in your kitchen and label them.

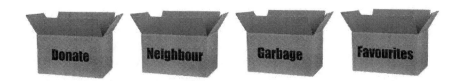

Fill the DONATE box with non-perishable foods that will go to a food bank or shelter. Make sure these are not open or past their expiry date.

The NEIGHBOUR box is for foods that might be open but still consumable. This box could go to a neighbour or to a friend; just make sure you get these items out of the house!

GARBAGE is for expired, rotten or open containers that cannot be donated or given away.

FAVOURITES is for those three food items you really love and will promise to keep tucked away for special occasions. You'll commit that these foods are not a part of your regular diet and are used only when you feel 100 percent in control of your cravings.

Nancy here: When I imagine losing a pound of fat, I visualize an entire foil-wrapped stick of butter coming off my thighs. A striking visual, no? How gross. And who is responsible for allowing that pound of butter to be there in the first place? Me!

So let's be clear. No one has done this to you but you. You have created where you are by eating the very crap you're about to take out of your kitchen. We get that this kitchen cleanse is tough but you can make it easy. Rip off the Band-Aid. And PLEASE celebrate doing this for you. You're worth it!

Step 1: Start with your pantry. Remove one item at a time. Choose which box that item will call its new home. As you place each item in the designated spot, take a deep breath and think to yourself, "I'm one step closer to my goal and I'm excited for this change!"

Pantry And Cupboards: Items On The Chopping Block

- Instant meals: ie. Mr. Noodle, Kraft Dinner, Hamburger Helper (bet you haven't heard that name in a while... or have you?)

- Canned meals: pasta, flavoured rice, pre-made soups, corn, pork and beans

- Canned fruits: with syrup

- Instant, flavoured oatmeal (plain is okay)

   Nancy here: When Michelle says plain, she means plain. That's straight up oatmeal. No sneaking in fake flavours, like peaches and cream or apple and cinnamon.

- Chips: do we really need to explain?

- Cookies: duh!

- Pastries: muffins and croissants (yup, sorry, these gotta go)

- Dried fruits: Don't panic because you thought these were healthy... they're better than many other snacks, but whole fruits are your best choice now as they are lower in sugar (per serving) and higher in that fill-you-up-fibre

- Candy and chocolate: (unless it's 85 percent or higher dark chocolate)

- Crackers: The following crackers are okay, but the rest go in the box!

Keep your: Mary's Crackers, Ryvita, Crunchmaster multigrain crackers, Enerjive Quinoa Skinny Crackers, Rye or Wasa crackers, Mediterranean Snack Food Co.

- Vegetable oils (including soy, canola sunflower and peanut)

- White flour

- Microwave popcorn

  Nancy here: once I learned what was in microwave popcorn, I went home that night and threw it all away! We're an air-popped only family now.

- Pop: just get it out of the house for now. This doesn't mean it's banned, but for now, keep it out of sight

- Alcohol (before you freak out, remember you get to keep three favourite items)

- Sugar and sugar-free Jello and puddings (packaged desserts)

- Sports drinks like Gatorade

Now, do the same with the contents of your fridge and freezer. Toss the stuff that won't propel you towards your goal, but rather slow down or completely halt your efforts.

Nancy here: I'm good at watching my food dollars and aware that others may be as well. You cannot find Your Weight Loss G-Spot without completing this task, though, so if you feel financially connected to the stuff in your fridge and freezer, you need to have a party and serve this food there. Or come up with another idea. Eating your way through it is NOT the solution and keeping it in your house isn't either. I have tried both and have lost the fight both times. I'm done losing and so are you!

Items To Ditch In Your Fridge And Freezer

- Concentrated juices: (Tang, frozen orange juice cans, any powdered juices you add water and sugar to)

- Any other juices: (other than those you juice yourself, unless it's pure prune… mmmmm, bet you can't wait for your prune juice!)

- Flavoured yogurts: (anything other than plain Greek yogurt must go)

- Frozen ready-made meals: (McCain's pizzas, Hot Pockets, Lean Cuisine, Michelina's etc.)

- Ice cream

- Jam and jellies

- Frozen breaded fish

- Breakfast sausages and other breakfast foods like hash browns

- Flavoured milks, including chocolate or sweetened alternative milks like sweetened soy, almond milks, etc.)

- Deli meats (unless they are organic)

- Cheese (you can keep low-fat mozzarella, Babybel, goat, Laughing Cow, cream cheese)

- Beer

- Syrups and sauces (maple syrup, sweet and sour and plum sauces)

Note: Condiments like ketchup, teriyaki sauce and BBQ sauce are super high in sugar. Keep these only if you feel like you can moderate their intake.

News Flash! Good Panty And Fridge/Freezer Items To Come!

Phew. Time to take a deep, cleansing breath. It feels like your pantry, fridge and freezer are empty, doesn't it? But the worst is over!

Nancy here: Don't panic. You're doing the right thing. Yes, it feels bad temporarily. So did the first time I had sex and now I'm writing about the G-Spot, for goodness sake.

Let me recap. You're going to make it way easier for yourself by clearing junky food from your home. Yay, you!

Think about it this way:

It's true that you're technically throwing away money, but remember, these foods are essentially garbage, so make peace with tossing garbage that will ultimately help you and your family in the long term. This money you spent buying that junk in the first place was a bad investment that's now impacting all your other life investments. Time to CUT BAIT!

Plus, keeping less processed foods in the kitchen will actually save you money down the road.

If there are any items you're unsure about because they're not on the list, ask yourself these questions to decide if that item is worth keeping or not:

1. Are there ingredients on the nutrients list that you can't pronounce? If so, toss it!

2. Does the item in its current form grow in the ground or on a plant or tree? If not, toss it.

3. If you were stranded on a deserted island and needed nourishment to survive, would this food fit the bill?

4. If you were looking to make a great first impression on your nutritionist friend (me), would you comfortably eat this in front of her? If not, you know what to do!

Step 2

You're so close to being done this part of the journey. Let's wrap it up! You now have 24 hours to move these boxes from your home to their pre-labeled designated areas.

Of course, you could stay G-Spot-less forever if you really wanted to, but I'm guessing you are ready for this next step.

Today is your day! It's go time! Celebrate your kitchen cleanse.

A note about Box 4: those favourites you kept behind for special occasions? Tuck them away. We're not there yet, so keep them out of sight for now.

C Is For Consume It!

GREAT news! Now, instead of getting rid of stuff, it's time to focus on what you get to eat that will get you closer to your G-Spot.

Consider the following foods denoted with a '*' as your staples. Think of staples as those foods that should be in your kitchen at all times. You can and should definitely add to this list, but make sure you have at least two or three items from each category handy at all times.

Use the following G-Friendly foods to construct your grocery list:

Protein

Choose lean and organic when available

- *Poultry: chicken, turkey*

- *Eggs*

- *Fish: salmon, cod, bass, haddock, halibut, perch, herring, tilapia, trout, mackerel, pike, sardines*

- *Greek yogurt (plain 0-2%)*

- *Cottage cheese (0-2%)*

- *Ricotta cheese (0-2%)*

- *Tuna (canned and fresh)*

- *Pheasant, quail, duck, goose*

- *Hen*

- *Game: bison, venison, elk*

- *Lean beef: flank, hamburger*

- *Pork (loin, chops)*

- *Lamb*

- *Shellfish: shrimp, oysters, scallops, mussels, crab, lobster*

- *Tofu*

- *Tempeh*

- *Soy burgers*

- **Hemp seeds (3 tbsp.) * I love the brand Manitoba Harvest Hemp*

- **Protein powders and bars (see below)*

Vegetables

Unlimited, so enjoy at every meal!

- *Bell pepper (red, orange, green)*

- *Asparagus*

- *Cabbage*

- *Brussels sprouts*

- *Okra*

- *Mushrooms*

- *Tomato*

- *Sprouts: alfalfa, sunflower, etc.*

- *Radish (including daikon)*

- *Parsnips*

- *Eggplant*

- *Jalapeno peppers*

- *Kohlrabi*

- *Sea vegetables: nori, kelp, wakame, kombu, dulse*

- *Zucchini*

- *Squash: acorn, butternut, spaghetti*

- *Shallots*

- *Turnips*

- **Sweet potatoes*

- *Yukon gold potatoes*

- *Water chestnuts*

- **Carrots*

- **Cauliflower*

- **Greens: kale, romaine, red lettuce, radicchio, spinach, mustard, watercress, dandelion, arugula, chicory*

- *Endive*

- *Beans (green and yellow)*

- *Endive*

- **Cucumber*

- *Fennel*

- **Onions*

- *Radishes*

- *Rutabagas*

- *Leeks*

- **Celery*

- *Peas: sugar snap, snow peas, split peas*

Fruits

Fresh is best!

- *Apples*

- *Pears*

- *Peaches*

- *Cherries*

- *Plums*

- *Cantaloupes*

- *Berries: raspberries, blueberries, blackberries, strawberries*

- *Bananas*

- *Watermelons*

- *Kiwis*

- *Mangoes*

- *Grapes*

- *Grapefruit*

- *Lemons*

- *Limes

- Oranges

- Nectarines

- Tangerines

- Apricots

- Papaya

- Pineapple

- Fresh figs

- Rhubarb

Oils

Healthy fats!

- *Extra virgin olive oil

- *Flax seeds and chia seeds

- Flax oil

- *Avocado

- Avocado oil

- Walnut oil

- *Olives (green or ripe)*

- *Sesame oil*

- **Coconut oil*

Whole Grains

- **Rice: brown rice, wild, brown basmati, rice noodles*

- *Millet*

- *Amaranth*

- *Corn*

- *Teff*

- **Quinoa*

- *Barley*

- *Whole wheat (pasta, breads, crackers)*

- *Rye*

- *Bulger*

- **Oat (steel cut oatmeal)*

- *Buckwheat*

- *Spelt*

What we love:

- Omega Nutrition Flax Seed oil

- Mary's Organic Crackers

- Stonemill and Ezekiel bread by Food for Life

- Bob's Red Mill wheat free oats

- *Kamut*

Dairy and Alternatives

- *Milk (1%-choose organic)*

- *Parmesan cheese*

- *Babybel (1)*

- *String cheese (1)*

- *Laughing cow (1)*

- *Feta (1oz), or goat cheese (1oz)*

- *Unsweetened almond milk*

- *Unsweetened rice milk*

- *Unsweetened coconut milk*

- *Unsweetened hemp or soy milk*

Nuts and Seeds

- **Almonds*

- **Hazelnuts*

- *Pecans*

- *Walnuts*

- *Sesame seeds (tahini)*

- *Sunflower seeds

- *Pumpkin seeds

- *Nut butters (from the above nuts and seeds)

Legumes

- *Kidney beans

- Lima beans

- Cannellini

- *Black beans

- Navy beans

- Mung beans

- Pinto beans

- *Garbanzo beans (chickpea)

- *Lentils

- Soy: edamame, TVP, miso

- *Hummus

- Soups made from the above beans

> **What we love:**
>
> - Eden Organic BPA free canned beans
>
> - Fontaine Sante hummus
>
> - Happy Planet and Amy's soups

Herbs, Spices and Condiments

Fresh or dried!

Herbs:

- *parsley, *basil, mint, bay, coriander, rosemary, fennel, *dill, chives, lemon balm, licorice, marigold, rosemary, sage, thyme, *oregano, etc.

Spices:

- *Cinnamon, cardamom, *ginger, *pepper, anise, cloves, nutmeg, saffron, *paprika, *cumin, chilli, curry, cayenne, *turmeric

Condiments:

- Horseradish, Sea salt (colour is key! Pick pinks and grays whenever possible), *Garlic, Gogi berries, Tamari (gluten free), *Vinegar: balsamic, apple cider, red wine

Sweeteners

- Agave nectar, *raw honey, stevia, *vanilla extract, almond extract

Beverages

- *Water

- Non-caffeinated herbal tea

- *Non-caffeinated green tea

Limited:

- organic coffee/ regular coffee, freshly juiced fruits, carbonated water

Anything on this list is fair game and will propel you forward towards your weight loss and healthy lifestyle goal.

Treats

The expectation is not that you are sugar-free for life. That's just not realistic.

But it is important to have a conversation about treats and how they play a role in your future. You will notice I used the word treat and not cheat. Let me say that again, treat versus (binge) cheat.

It doesn't matter if you long for sugar or salt, consider the list above your Bible. For now, other foods not on the list are DENIED.

There are however a few packaged items and protein snacks that are acceptable.

Here are a few suggestions.

Michelle's List of Healthy Packaged Snacks

- *Square snacks*

- *Fontain Sante hummus (the roasted garlic flavour is my favourite!)*

- *Sasha and company Organic Buckwheat Snacks*

- *PC Guacamole seasoning mix*

- *Lara Bars*

- *Quest Protein Bars, specifically Coconut Cashew*

- *Simply Bars*

- *Genuine Health Fermented Proteins +protein bars*

- *LundBerg rice cakes with almond butter*

- *Kind Bars*

- *Three Farmers Roasted Chick Peas*

- *Protein Powders blended into a delicious smoothie (see below)*

Protein Powders

We live life at an insane pace, so I'm a huge fan of some of the clean sources of protein powders on the market. There are many types of powders available. Some are junk (filled with sugars, artificial sweeteners, preservatives, food colouring and more), but there are others that are simple and contain good quality ingredients.

Tip: At times I have clients cringe at the cost of some clean protein powders. If you decide to use them, include these in your overall cost of living. They are replacing or being used in addition to other foods and should therefore be part of your total grocery bill.

Before deciding if protein powders are right for you or not, keep in mind the following points:

- Nothing replaces whole, fresh foods—even clean protein powders.

- There are many different types of protein powders. The most available forms come in whey, rice, pea, hemp and soy.

- The type of protein powder you choose depends on a few factors including your:

Taste buds

Allergies

Food sensitivities

Cost

Lifestyle

For example, I will often recommend a whey-based protein powder for individuals who are doing resistance–based strength training. Whey is an extremely absorbable form of protein and aids in quicker recovery after training.

Or for those people who might be sensitive to dairy, a vegan-based protein powder is a better option.

Protein Powders at a Glance

*My advice is to pick up small sample packets of as many options as possible so you can decide on your favourite before committing to a large tub.

TYPE OF PROTEIN	PROTEIN (G) PER SERVING	PRIMARY TYPE OF PROTEIN
VEGA SPORT	1 serving= 25 g	Pea, rice, hemp
VEGA ONE	1 serving = 15 g	Pea, hemp, rice
GARDEN OF LIFE: RAW PROTEIN	1 serving = 18 g	Rice
SUNWARRIOR (RICE OR VEGAN)	1 serving = 17 g	Rice, pea, cranberry, hemp
MANITOBA HEMP PRO	4 tbsp. = 21 g	Hemp
OMEGA NUTRITION PUMPKIN SEED POWDER	3 tbsp.=20 g	Pumpkin seeds
GENUINE HEALTH FERMENTED VEGAN PROTEINS +	1 serving= 20 g	Pea, rice, potato, hemp
NUTRIBIOTIC RICE PROTEIN	1 serving = 11 g	Rice
NORTH COAST NATURALS	1 serving = 24 g	Whey
LEAN FIT COMPLETE GREEN PROTEIN	1 serving = 18 g	Pea, hemp, rice

Protein Bars

I'm often asked about protein bars and where they fit into a healthy diet. The reality is that most bars are extremely high in sugars and despite their protein content, are just not good options for most people trying to lose fat. There are, however, a few bars I have found that are okay to eat once in a while as an on-the-go protein-rich snack option.

BAR	PROTEIN (G)	SUGAR (G)	WE LIKE	WATCH OUT
SIMPLY BAR (PEANUT BUTTER)	15	1	High fibre, low sugar, high protein	
QUEST BAR (COCONUT CASHEW)	20	1 + 5 g sugar alcohols	High fibre, low sugar, high protein	
GENUINE HEALTH FERMENTED VEGAN PROTEINS +	13	9	The fermented ingredients help support the growth of good bacteria in our intestinal system	
CLIFF BAR (PEANUT BUTTER)	11	21		High in sugar for those trying to lose fat
LUNA PROTEIN	12	15		Sugar too high
KIND BARS	6	6	Clean, natural ingredients	A little low in protein

Nancy here: Michelle has explained the importance of getting enough protein, whether or not you choose to supplement with a bar or a powder. Through my work with Michelle, I know that I need to do whatever it takes to consume enough protein. With my insane schedule, this can make finding the time to eat protein feel like I'm on The Amazing Race. My solution? I buy Quest Protein Bars in bulk. Literally. I have two in my car, two in my workbag, and two in my overnight travel bag. Why? To eliminate any excuse for me to grab a cookie/sweet sugar devil of a treat, when what I really need is a protein fix.

I also travel with a hand blender, a large "flexi" cup and my morning protein shake ingredients so my routine is the same wherever I wake up. This may sound insane to you—but it works for me. Be patient and figure out what works for you.

Either way, many of the same principles that you learned about label reading above apply when you're choosing protein powders and bars. Keep the sugars low, skip the artificial sweeteners and be aware of harmful preservatives and food colourings—all are toxic to a healthy G-Spot!

You've learned that real food is the right choice, and you're only beginning the G-Spot experience when you're clear about what real is.

And now, all this talk about food is making me thirsty....

D Is For Drink: Water!

Unofficially, in my mind, the fourth macronutrient, after carbohydrates, fats and protein, is water.

We've all heard it a million times. I know and you know, we all need to drink our water—but do you know why?

I'll give it to you straight:

- As you begin to lose fat, toxins will be released from your cells. If they are not flushed out properly, "toxins may interact with our hormones and cause increased fat storage and inability to burn fat."

- Water also hydrates our brain, allowing us to feel more energized and positive. This is key to ensuring healthy meals are on the table and workouts are completed!

- Water helps to keep us full. Often, we think we're hungry when we're really just thirsty and ultimately this can lead to consuming unnecessary calories.

- What many people don't know is that water actually slightly increases the metabolic rate.

Yes, you read that correctly—when you drink water, the rate at which you burn calories at rest is increased. It's time to get on board with water if you aren't already!

How much you ask? Aim for approximately 2 litres per day; this is equal to about 8 cups. If you are active, you need more.

FAQ

Q. Does tea and coffee count towards my 2 litres for the day?

A. No. Black tea and coffee are diuretics and will actually draw water out of your system, so make sure you have your 2 litres minimum in addition to these.

Q. Does the water found in the fruit and vegetables from my food list count towards the 2 Litres per day?

A. No. Please consume 2 litres of fresh water in addition to any fluids found in foods.

Q. If I work out, do I need more than 2 litres per day?

A. Yes. Ideally, you would replace any water lost during exercise. Please ensure you are getting minimum .5-1L (or more depending on the intensity) extra of water when active.

Consuming adequate amounts of water, good quality carbohydrates, proteins and healthy fats will most certainly set you on the right path for weight loss success.

Treats, Not Cheats

I know you're dying to read this part! I can read your mind.

Moving forward through this book and journey, a clear-cut plan will be built by you that identifies how to design a personal treat boundary that not only works for you but will help drive you towards reducing cravings and losing fat effectively.

We need to take back control and this means eliminating sugar for a short period of time.

Nancy here: Haven't we have had enough "last suppers" for a country? Consider this already DONE!

Skip the "I'm starting my diet tomorrow" binge or "just one last slice of cake and then I'm done with sugar." You are done now, right now. You've got this!

And now, it's my story time. I call this one "Car Cookies".

Usually when I "diet," after a few days, I get on a roll. It's an awesome feeling. I feel lighter and I think, "Hey, I really think I'm going to lose the weight this time!

And then I go grocery shopping. Feeling superior, I walk the cookie aisle. I think "I've got this", and I decide that because I have such excellent self-control I can handle buying cookies as a special treat for my kids when they get home from school.

And then guess what happens? The moment I am alone with the cookies (or when I decide the cookies are so special they need to ride home in the front seat with me), I eat the entire box.

ON THE WAY HOME.

Exchange Nancy's cookies with your BIGGEST temptation (ice cream, chocolate, etc.), and the end result will be the same. That's why you aren't ready to go treat shopping yet. It's not time. You're in learning mode on how to make good choices.

Don't believe me? Try this. Buy your favourite food vice with a plan of moderation. Test yourself.

And if you have more than one serving every four days, start back at Chapter 1 of this book because you've missed a couple of key points and you're not ready to get on the G-Spot ride just yet.

Once you have completed the above-required steps (cleaning out your kitchen and restocking it with healthy choices), use the next chapter as a guide for healthier treat selections if you chose to include these in your plan—but remember, not yet—we're still getting to this!

Chapter 4: Keys to G (we know this one was a doozy!)

- Skip unhealthy products like trans fats and hydrogenated oils. They only add to your waistline, plus they're inflammatory and overall, no good for you!

- Good fats help protect your cells, provide energy, help raise the good, HDL cholesterol and help speed up fat loss

- Aim for approximately 20g protein per meal (3 per day) and 5-10g protein per snack (2 per day)

- Avoid poor cuts of meat like bacon and deli meats

- Choose lean, clean protein sources like poultry, salmon, plain Greek yogurt and protein powders

- Bag the junk and restock from the lists provided. This is it! Time to get down and dirty and make it count

- Drink water! It's a must in my book if you are trying to drop the pounds. It keeps you energized and helps with fat and toxin flushing. Aim for approximately 2 litres per day

WANT MORE HELP?

Want to learn more? We have created a free workbook to go along with this book. You will also find a list of great books, websites and other valuable bonus resources to will help you dive deeper!

Get access to your free bonus resources at
http://bonus.weightlossgspot.com/

5

A LITTLE TO THE LEFT

Hey, it's Nancy back! Are you ready to talk treats?

You're either reading this book and you've come this far with us because you want to have the best life EVER—or maybe you just really want to know where your Weight Loss G-Spot is!

I'm assuming you're craving the best life ever. For me, that means being fully present every single day. It means enjoying moments. It means connecting with others and relishing in sharing amazing experiences.

But when you stop to consider our North American society and relate it to our idea of our best life, you quickly realize that many of the moments we treasure revolve around food: lavish dinners out, cozy family breakfasts, birthday parties with cake and ice cream, barbecues with beer and ribs.

As you read this, you've gotta be wondering how the heck to make these transforming lifestyle changes in a culture that often feels like it's tap dancing through a never-ending buffet line.

Here's the thing. Our culture isn't going to change anytime soon, so it's up to you. We're here to empower you with some tips and tricks to enable you to enjoy group settings so you can continue living your life fully while respecting your decision to put your health and your Weight Loss G-Spot first. Time to lead with your need!

We'll want to play around in three areas to set you up for success:

First, tips and tricks to handling group settings with food, otherwise known as The Food Orgy.

Then, how to go about treating yourself when you want a treat…

Michelle here: Within moderation!

Third, great recipes you can make and contribute to events (as hostess gifts, dessert for after dinner, etc.) to give you options in any situation.

Michelle here: Nancy and I have included a few of our favourite treats that are also secretly healthy.

The Food Orgy

It's crazy how often we're put into a food orgy situation. In my career, I'd say 95 percent of the meetings and sessions I attend include platters and trays, overflowing with food. Other than the odd fruit or veggie platter, this stuff is on-site prepared stomach entertainment: items include lots of highly processed sauces, simple carbs like pasta dishes or premade sandwiches, and dessert trays that instantly make my mouth water.

Recently I was running a two-day Intentional Leaders session in Regina, Saskatchewan. Our 8 a.m., in-room breakfast service included a tray of 40 cake-like finger desserts… for 18 of us! You and I both know that if this is the way you're starting your day, you're a goner!

Michelle here: remember when we discussed the cookie? Turn back to Chapter 4 if you need a reminder of the impact sugar has on our energy levels!

On the other hand, I know specific companies and hotels that do a fantastic job providing healthy(er) (and tasty) alternatives. In fact, this is where I sampled my first quinoa cookie!

Here's what I've noticed happening more and more in the last six months. Session participants, men and women alike, are starting to bring their own food.

I LOVE IT! I recently shared a chat with a participant (after commenting on the protein bar she had at her setting, beside a container of almonds and a second container of apple slices) about her decision to bring her own food. She said after some life changes she made, it's the right thing for her. End of story. How's that for owning a decision?

Michelle here: Love this! I love when people can make a good decision for themselves and make peace with it. The more you fight it and feel sorry for yourself, the longer and harder it will be to find Your Weight Loss G-Spot. Trust me on this one.

For me, I know that once the prospect of the food orgy is introduced, my head wanders to the orgy climax. My climax fantasy includes all other meeting partakers looking the other way while I gorge and grab more than my fair share of X (and depending on the buffet, X changes).

Bottom line: if I even consider circling the food orgy display, the feeling of control slips from my hands like an over-lubed dildo.

Doesn't matter if it's a work meeting food tray, a wedding buffet table or a box of Halloween candy, you know your food orgy of choice. Time to reimagine the climax so you'll still be able to participate and be there!

Here are 11 tips Michelle and I give clients in preparation of being in close proximity to a food orgy area:

1. Drink LOTS of water before entering. How much, you ask? FILL YOURSELF with water!

2. Eat a nutritious meal or snack before you go. Arrive with a full stomach. After all, you're there for the meeting or celebration or to catching up, so focus on that!

3. When asked why you're not scarfing down food like it's your last meal, simply say, "I just ate," or "There was food at my last meeting," or "I didn't realize there would be lunch here." That will shush the food pushers up for at least a few hours.

4. Bring food with you. If it's a meeting, bring a soft, cloth lunch bag with foods you actually like versus foods that make you say, "Ugh, they get to eat that while I gnaw on carrots?" Or if it's a dinner or get-together at a friend's house, offer to bring a dessert or appetizer you'll look forward to.

5. Stand away from the food so you're not smack-dab in firing range. When you can't see the temptation, you're not inclined to munch unconsciously!

6. Go in with parameters. If you are choosing to have a treat, then choose ahead of time what it will be and how much you'll have. Setting these guidelines ahead of time makes you more likely to abide by your own rules. For me, this rule is the game changer.

When I do this, I am successful. I don't do this, and I might as well put a bib on and yell, "Food-eating contest!"

7. Pick your poison. We mentioned this before. If you have previously decided to have a treat, pick your favourite and not just munch on junk because it's simply there. Make sure what you eat is your MOST favourite. For me, it's gotta be at least an 8 out of 10.

8. Chew gum.

9. Keep a drink (water, tea or coffee) in your hand. This will make holding a giant plate of food more difficult.

10. Fill up on the good stuff first. Fill a plate with veggies and fruit, shrimp, olives, guacamole etc. Most likely, you won't feel as hungry after that.

11. Self-talk. Sometimes it's as simple as asking yourself, "Will this food propel me towards or away from my goal? "If the answer is away, take a breather, go for a walk and give it a minute, then decide. If a closed-ended question will make your "other inner voice" freak out, then a question is not for you. Here's what I say: "Nance. You have got this. You are worth this. Eating food that nourishes your body makes your heart sing and your positive head chatter win. Take care of you like only you can. I love you."

> **Tip:** Make a copy of the 11 tips. Keep it handy, like in your bra. Read it before starting your day, going to a meeting or arriving at a networking event.

Yes, it's third person. It's my speech. It works for me. RIGHT NOW prepare your speech. Consider it the most successful pickup line you'll ever use.

How about when you're at a sit-down dinner, or a place where you feel pressure to partake in the food? Here are 10 tips and tricks:

1. Liken the thought of overeating to drunkenness. How appropriate would this be at the table? What would be appropriate? How would that make you feel? How do you plan to think of it this way?

2. Savour each bite. Chew slowly. You didn't have to cook it, so celebrate!

3. You know what your body needs. Scoop more of the good stuff on your plate and bend a rule with a half-scoop of a treat food IF you must.

4. Put your fork down between bites. This will allow your stomach time to fill up and signal to your brain you are full.

5. Eat the protein and veggie portion of the meal first. If you're still hungry, have a small portion of the starch.

6. Limit your alcohol. Too much to drink equals extra calories, but it also lowers your inhibitions and your ability to make sound decisions in the moment. Just like in college!

7. Buddy up. Share a dessert with your BFF or husband/boyfriend. When none of these support people are around? Cut the dessert in half and focus on your half of the plate. When it's done, push it away, cover it in pepper (to remove the possible temptation) and walk away from the table. Always have an exit strategy!

8. Treat appetizers as part of the meal. If the option is good, like soup or salad, fill up on this because the next part of the meal might not be as G-Spot friendly.

9. Ask ahead of time. Don't be afraid to inquire about the meal selection for that night. Simply say you wanted to be able to bring something to contribute or perhaps you have a food sensitivity you need to be mindful of. Either way, if this person is a friend or family they will be happy to give you this information. Why? So then you can create a plan or vision! Here's what I'm facing, here's what I'll eat, here's how I'll handle what I won't, etc.

10. Know that not every meal is going to be perfect. So instead, keep your diet 90 percent clean when you're home so you have a little more leeway when it comes to social events.

A food orgy can get pretty crazy. There are just so many options everywhere and it's easy to get caught up in the feeding frenzy. But just like from sex, I'm looking for more from my food than gluttonous quantities. I want quality. I want nourishment. That's my choice.

Treating Yourself When You Want A Treat

"I REALLY WANT A TREAT!" That's what my head says—over and over and over like a whiny child eying the candy beside their exhausted parent in the grocery checkout line.

But this is not the time to indulge in a treat! This is the time to do ANYTHING but give your food orgy-loving thoughts a treat. Why? Because you're not thinking straight. You are over thinking, you are obsessively thinking, you are tunnel-treat-vision thinking.

When this happens, set a timer. You heard me... a timer. Set it for 20 minutes.

Take 20 minutes to connect to what's important, to think about your vision board, to go over your plan. Breathe, pause, call a friend and regroup.

In 20 minutes, you get to make a decision. Earn the treat. If it's helpful, take a picture of this paragraph on your smartphone and read it ANYTIME you need to. I'm serious. DO IT!

Rule of thumb: aim for a treat to contain no more than 150 calories per serving and under 10g of sugar.

I'm back, it's Michelle and am going to jump in here to walk you through the ins and outs of treats!

Here are a few other tools I suggest to clients when they are craving:

First, ask yourself, "Will this treat propel me towards or away from my goal?" This simply helps you to reconnect with your weight loss goal. Sometimes this can get lost in a craving haze.

If that doesn't do the trick, try what I like to call The 3 Stops. It's a good way to help delay giving into a craving.

- Have a big glass of water to fill you up

- Brush your teeth! This helps change the chemistry in your mouth and gets you away from the kitchen

- Move it! Run up and down your stairs for two minutes or go for a 5-minute walk. Anything that will get your heart rate going and your serotonin levels (your happy chemical) up.

So next time you are faced with a craving situation, try the above, they work. Cross my heart.

So what exactly, is a treat?

According to the all-knowing Google, a treat is "an event or item that is out of the ordinary and gives great pleasure."

Based on this definition, choose wisely (from your favourites) and choose appropriately (limit to a few per week).

Okay, so you earned a treat. How many treats do you get to have in a week?

Typically if you are female and have more than 10 pounds to lose, I'm asking to you stick to 2 to 4 treats per week. This might not seem like a lot right now, but if you plan for them and choose your favourites, you will really learn to appreciate them!

My Favourite Treats

- Dark chocolate 70% or higher (I LOVE the Endangered Species chocolate 88% brand)

- 4-5oz glass of wine

- Fresh fruit dipped in Greek yogurt (ideally plain yogurt but if you have sweetened, please have a small portion)

- Simply Protein chips

- Sugar-free iced coffee made with unsweetened almond or cashew milk, cinnamon and ice cubes (blend if you'd like)

- 2 cups popcorn (preferably homemade and drizzled with olive oil, spices and sea salt)

- 1 to 2 cookies (see Rule of thumb box for guideline and consider purchasing only 1 or 2 cookies [about 100-150 calories] instead of the whole box. I like the GoGo Quinoa cookies!)

- So Delicious coconut ice cream (found in many local grocery and health food stores)

- Raw cacao nibs drizzled with raw honey and blueberries

Recipes For You To Try At Home

We've compiled a small list of our favourite treats and desserts for you to create in your kitchen if you'd rather not face the temptations in the grocery store.

This is not an exhaustive list, but a reference for you compare other recipes against. You'll notice that all the recipes below contain very little sugar; this is key to preventing cravings.

Treat Recipes

Mouth-Watering Macaroons

Oven-Free Nut Butter Energy Bars

No-Bake Banana Chocolate Protein Bars

Almond Joy Bites

Mouth-Watering Macaroons

- 1 ½ tablespoons of sugar

- ½ teaspoon of vanilla extract

- 1 cup of unsweetened coconut

- 2 egg whites, whisked to frothy

Directions

Add 1 ½ tablespoons of sugar

Add a touch of vanilla extract or almond extract for flavour and cinnamon if you'd like!

Then add 1 cup of coconut (sweetened or unsweetened; personally I opt for unsweetened and add more vanilla when I make these, or drizzle them with dark chocolate)

Then drop by the spoonful on parchment paper.

Bake at 375 for 15 to 20 minutes, or until they get a nice light brown top coat

Oven-Free Nut Butter Power Bars

- ½ cup agave nectar

- 1 ½ cup nut butter (peanut, almond or cashew)

- 3 cups wheat-free oatmeal

- 2 scoops vanilla protein powder

- 2 tbsp. coconut oil

- ½ cup dried cranberry

- ½ cup slivered almonds

- ½ cup pumpkin seeds

Directions

Warm agave, coconut and nut butter in sauce pan until ingredients are soft enough to easily combine when mixed. Remove from heat.

Add oatmeal and protein powder and mix well. Then add dried fruits, almonds and seeds. Mix well.

Press into 9 inch square pan. Let cool in the fridge and cut into squares.

No-Bake Banana Chocolate Protein Bars

Now you can quickly and easily make your own protein bars at home! This no-bake recipe takes high-quality protein powder and combines it with wholesome, real food ingredients to create a delicious protein bar to power your day. Store these in your freezer, then simply allow to defrost for a few minutes before enjoying. This recipe makes 10 bars.

- 1 cup vanilla protein powder (see chapter 4 for protein options)

- ¼ cup coconut flour

- 2 mashed bananas

- ½ cup coconut milk

- ¼ cup water (more if needed)

- 1 teaspoon vanilla extract

- 2 tbsp. mini chocolate chips (or substitute raw cacao nibs or nuts)

- 1 oz. dark chocolate (70% cocoa or higher)

- 1 teaspoon coconut oil

Directions

In a medium bowl, combine the protein powder and coconut flour.

In another medium bowl, mash the bananas. Add coconut milk, water and vanilla and mix until smooth. Add the dry ingredients and mix until fully combined. If the batter is dry, add a few more drops of water. Mix in the chocolate chips.

Line a freezer-safe plate with wax paper. Form the dough into 10 bars. Place on the wax paper and put in the freezer for 20 minutes.

In a double boiler over medium-low heat (if you don't have a double boiler, make your own by placing a small saucepan directly in a skillet containing a few tablespoons of water), melt the dark chocolate.

Remove the bars from the freezer and drizzle or dip in the melted dark chocolate.

Return to the freezer for 10 minutes until the chocolate has hardened.

Source: Bianca Schaefer. Mississauga Adventure Boot Camp

Almond Joy Bites

Ingredients

- 14 dates

- ¼ cup almond butter

- 2 heaping tbsp. unsweetened coconut flakes

- 2 tbsp. cacao powder

- 2 tbsp. chia seeds

- 2 tbsp. raw honey

- handful of enjoy life mini chocolate chips

Directions

Pulse everything except the chocolate chips together in a food processor until well incorporated.

Stir in chocolate chips.

Roll into balls, place on a large plate or sheet tray and refrigerate.

Keep in the fridge until ready to eat.

Notes

- Makes about 12 balls.

- Recipe from joyoushealth.com

Chapter 5: Keys to G

- You now have the power and control to define for yourself what you consider a treat. Get clear on this. The difference between a treat and a binge MUST be clear before you have a treat.

- What I now know: With practice, a real treat is no longer food for me. A treat is something that makes me grin authentically, something I can enjoy it for a while, like a good book, a walk on the beach on a gorgeous day, or some great laughing and play time with friends. Know what you want a treat to feel like, and go from there.

6

TRIGGER THIS!

It's Nancy again, here to discuss an issue we all have difficulty confronting—those trying, troublesome, tricky triggers.

Here it is... the confrontation you've been waiting for. It's time for you to come clean, to admit to and reveal your personal kryptonite.

It's time to reveal your trigger!

Here are some textbook definitions of the word **trigger:**

noun:

1. a small projecting tongue in a firearm that, when pressed by the finger, actuates the mechanism that discharges the weapon;

2. a device, as a lever, the pulling or pressing of which releases a detent or spring;

3. anything, as an act or event, that serves as a stimulus and initiates or precipitates a reaction or series of reactions.

verb (used with object):

1. to initiate or precipitate (a chain of events, scientific reaction, psychological process, etc.). e.g. Their small protest triggered a mass demonstration.

2. to fire or explode (a gun, missile, etc.) by pulling a trigger or releasing a triggering device: e.g. He accidentally triggered his rifle.

Key words that stand out to me from the definitions above:

- Fire

- Explode

- Reaction

- Psychological process

- Weapon

Now, here's our personal definition of a trigger, as it applies to this book:

Specific things that seem to set you off—more than usual—to sabotage your healthy plan for eating.

Let's start with why we need to identify our triggers.

Imagine for a moment that you're driving in your neighbourhood. Every time you round the corner, four houses from your home, your car gets a flat tire. Every. Single. Time.

UGH!

How does this nightmarish Groundhog Day-like experience affect you?

Lots! It takes time away from the stuff you need to get done, wastes your money (because you have to keep to fixing or replacing your tire) and creates dread about your drive home (you might even develop an anxiety of what's waiting around the corner). Yet, you keep on doing the same thing, every day.

You don't take another route home. You don't consider alternative options to get you from point A to B. You don't park the car on the side of the road so you can figure out what the heck may be causing you to get a flat tire every day.

I'm sure you'll agree with me when I say this is absolutely absurd thinking.

But wait a second. Let's think about the way we treat food, and our blindness and ignorance towards our food triggers. They've been affecting our judgment for so long, they've become just the way it is, and we don't even consider taking a different path.

Reread the last sentence. Note especially the word "just" as in "just the way it is". For the record, I'm not into the idea of "just"; in fact, I've removed the word from my vocabulary. It drives me nuts when I hear people say, "It's just not for me," or "Never mind; it's just me."

In my opinion, the word "just" can belittle. It sends the message to others (and to ourselves) that it's not important. Part of this stems from how we've used it in casual conversation versus what the word actually means.

Bottom line: be cognizant on how you use the word "just", specifically for yourself. Notice if it's an excuse: i.e. "just the way it is" and how you use it to prioritize your needs with others.

Consider when to rephrase and step into YOU and own what you believe! "Just" doesn't cut it anymore. If you're done with "just" in your life—if it's NOT okay for you to "just" do anything anymore—keep reading.

With all that being said, let's talk triggers.

Here's a fact: triggers are going to pop up in every life situation, not only with food habits. The key is how you handle the trigger.

First, though, you need to be super clear of what your particular triggers are, specifically for food and eating habits.

My guess is that some of these triggers are so second nature for you that you aren't even aware they exist. Simply, it's just what you do and you don't even stop to think any differently!

Here's an example. One of my friends grew up eating berries for dessert—with sugar sprinkled on top. She assumed that this is how everyone eats berries, because it's all she's ever known. It was just the way it is for her!

Identification Time!

Let's play in two areas—your feelings and your actions—to explore what trigger points you may have. We're starting with your feelings.

Feelings

Feelings are characterized by an emotion, state or response. When we're young, we learn which feelings people don't necessarily want to see. This includes emotions like sadness, frustration, and disappointment.

We learn to "suck it up, buttercup," and that "no one likes a sourpuss." Or how about this gem: "Turn that frown upside down?"

We quickly acquire an understanding of which feelings others prefer to see and what happens when they appear.

"My Mom likes it when I smile," for example, or "My teacher says lazy kids are bad," or "My Dad gets angry when we play in the garden." Through our early years, we start to tailor our expressions by concealing feelings that draw negative responses and work to enhance or turn up feelings that others seem to prefer to see. Regardless of our natural instinct, we have been trained to provide expected behaviour responses to situations, responses that display the appropriate, approved feeling.

Fast forward from today to your childhood 19 plus years ago (feel free to place yourself accordingly on the age spectrum!) and think about this.

Most of our thinking is shaped during the first 16 years of our life, and our learned responses to our feelings may be similar to what was illustrated in the flat tire anecdote. We agreed, didn't we, that this type of thinking is absurd?

Surprising? Maybe. But it's true.

We want to focus on identifying your triggers and what habits you have created as a result. And hey! The best part is that you're reading this book to reprogram yourself to where you'd prefer to be.

But before you can adjust your thinking habits, you need to be hyperaware of exactly what you are feeling. Let me explain this with a story.

The Game Changer

I was facilitating a session about using Intentional Communication with Coaching. To consistently practice Intentional Communication, there are important skills you need to apply. These include what we call Level 2 listening (listening for both facts and feelings in conversation), using your instincts, confirming (with a rephrase) what the other person has said, and acknowledging the feelings the person has shared (verbally or otherwise). We were almost to the end of Day One (of four days), when a male participant in the room raised his hand and said, "I get it. I really do. Listening for feelings and acknowledging them is clearly part of both the communication and the coaching process and if I am to get better at communicating, I must do this. I'm watching the other participants do this so easily, but I don't have the feeling words they do. I literally know four feelings: happy, sad, frustrated and angry. What do I do?"

Two other male participants in the room nodded in agreement. And then there was some heckling. (An aside: this was a great group who brought a sense of humour to their learning and they were not afraid to be vulnerable—my favourite kind of people!) I asked for permission to challenge the three guys to create a master list of 60 "emotion and feelings words" after the dinner event that evening. The rest of the group thought this was a riot! That awesome trio then went out and enjoyed some bevvies while making their way through this challenge. The next morning, they brought "feelings words" written on cocktail napkins. Yes, there were some cheating spin-offs like: "joy," then "joyful," then, "joyous," even "joy-errific," but overall it was a thorough list. When I asked what their take away from the exercise was, the recap included: a better grasp on how large the "feeling rainbow" was, a clear "go to" list of words that would help better connect with others and finally—and most satisfying for me—the male that initiated the conversation said, "This is a game-changer for me."

The reason I share this with you: Be aware of the feelings that are linked to your food triggers—and you'll find the game-changer!

If you can't label or acknowledge what the feeling is, how the heck can you both be with it AND shift it?

Before we begin The Game Changer exercise, here is a list of 56 feelings (note that there is a combination of feelings listed). In my opinion, there are no good or bad feelings. Just being aware of your feelings is the first step in taking action.

Instructions for The Game Changer exercise:

1. Put a star beside the feelings you enjoy having.

2. Circle the ones that make you uncomfortable (when you feel this emotion, your reaction is to get away from it, tune it out or block it).

*Please list any feelings we've missed but you think you'd like on the list.

THE GAME CHANGER EXERCISE

Confident	Courageous	Peaceful	Happy
Alive	Playful	Calm	Sensitive
Angry	Depressed	Sad	Anxious
Nervous	Exhilarated	Energized	Afraid
Glad	Friendly	Surprised	Thankful
Pride	Sympathetic	Hurt	Stressed
Shocked	Generous	Relief	Love
Sadness	Embarrassed	Amused	Doubtful
Frustrated	Empathy	Bored	Affectionate
Envy	Guilt	Shame	Irritated
Optimistic	Eager	Shy	Worry
Longing	Bliss	Helplessness	Fear
Disappointed	Spite	Vengeful	Rapture
Eagerness	Uneasy	Torment	Agitated
_____	_____	_____	_____

Reflection time.

Here, we'll reflect on a couple of feelings you placed a star beside and a couple you circled.

But first, read my explanations below so you understand how your response may have been formed.

Reflecting on the feeling words you placed a star besides, what allows you to comfortably be with these?

For example: Pride. When I feel proud, I actually feel like I beam from the inside. If I have worked at something to achieve it or support someone else to meet their goal through my skill set, pride runs through my veins like a warm glow. It's a glorious, alive feeling that reminds me what's important to me.

Reflecting on the feelings words you circled, describe what happens when "the feel" starts and then consider literally, in steps, what you do to avoid feeling the feel.

_____

_____

_____

Let's use "isolated" as another example. If I go from a full day at work or a week with lots on my social calendar to a quiet Saturday, the time by myself can unbalance me energy-wise and I'm pushed toward the kitchen (to use food to TEMPORARILY change what I am feeling inside).

As you can see from the two examples, the second example actually begins explaining the why: defending it, detailing it. If there were real

> **AUTHOR NOTE:** IF THIS IS HARD, THERE'S A FEELING HERE FOR YOU. PLEASE STAY HERE. THINK ABOUT IT. SHAKE IT UP. FIGURE IT OUT. WE ARE WRITING THIS BOOK—AND YOU'RE READING THIS BOOK—BECAUSE YOU DESERVE TO FEEL YOUR LIFE MOMENTS VERSUS "FUNCTION-LIKE" WITHIN YOUR LIFE. YOU'VE GOT THIS. OWN THIS.

comfort in this feeling, there would be no explanation required. With the pride example, I expressed my response through my language. But with the isolation example, I defended it and used an explanation to attempt to support the excuse about why I was eating.

Learn To Feel Through Coaching

There's a reason the above note was in CAPS. It's extra important. For lots of us, the eating isn't about the food, it's about the hole we're filling inside of us. If you don't figure the feeling/emotional stuff out, the eating will continue. I know this first-hand.

DOWNLOAD YOUR FREE WORKBOOK

Remember to download the free Workbook. We created PDF's so you can print them out and use as you are working your way through the book. This will aid greatly in your success!

Get access to your free bonus resources at
http://bonus.weightlossgspot.com/

Reflection on feelings you starred:

Feeling: _____

_____

_____

_____

Feeling: _____

_____

_____

_____

Feeling: _____

_____

_____

_____

Reflection on Feelings you circled:

Feeling: _____

_____

_____

Feeling: _____

_____

_____

_____

Feeling: _____

_____

_____

_____

Again, to make this easier for you, download the free workbook where you can fill in your answers from this link:

http://bonus.weightlossgspot.com/

Looking at the answers you gave, summarize how the above impacts:

   a) What you chose to eat when your starred feelings come up:

_____

_____

_____

b) Habits that you have created with food (circled feeling) for immediate gratification versus BEing with yourself and your feeling:

_____

_____

_____

i.e. I have a 3 p.m. lull. I say to myself, "I've made it this far… what can I fill myself with for rest-of-the-day energy?"

Here's a little bit of personal sharing. Some people have specific emotions that they directly relate to eating; they feel "this" and find food immediately (to distract from pain, discomfort, etc.).

For example, I had a very busy client. She would consistently eat healthy foods all day. Then when she went to wind down for the evening in her favourite way, watching television, she would eat a large bag of chips with a cola! The drastic change of her pace and stress level from GO GO GO to STOP was a jump too significant for her to deal with—so she created a food spike to get through it.

> *Michelle here: I always say that everyone is on a diet until about 3 p.m. Up until then we are happy, content on "the wagon." Then mid-afternoon, S%#t hits the fan, life gets hectic again and it's time to find solace in other things like eating. If this is you, you are neither alone nor strange. But it is time to break the habit and find joy elsewhere!*

The Wagon

I've been thinking a lot about the term "bandwagon" lately. As in:

"I'm on the wagon."

"I'm off the wagon."

"I hate the wagon."

and my personal favourite,

"I am dragging by a thread behind the wagon."

I went online to get some ideas about the term bandwagon. The term has morphed from the original "on the water cart," which was a device once used to transfer drunk and disorderlies to a location to sober up and has now evolved to either mean abstaining from a bad habit; or participating in a night of binge drinking and then sobering up the next day.

So we seem to have linked the wagon with behaving badly (too much food, too much drink, too much consumption) or with needing to change a bad habit.

But wait a minute. Who actually owns the wagon? Hmmmm. That would be you! And you control whether you're on it, off it or hanging behind it by a thread.

My suggestion: consider the wagon. Create your own wagon to be what you want and need it to be so it fits the role required to get you to YOUR G-Spot.

Picture your personal wagon as a jalopy. It's an oldie, a bare-bones, three-sided box of wood on wheels that would only be tolerable for a short ride into town, something Laura and Pa would have travelled in on Little House on the Prairie. No wonder you're not lasting on this wagon!

We shared a great visual exercise with you in Chapter 2. Using those same skills, get clear, really clear, on what YOUR WAGON to YOUR G-SPOT looks and feels like. There's a lot better chance of you staying on the ride if you actually like what (or who) you're riding!

Personally, I couldn't pinpoint any one or two emotions that provoked me to eating excessively because I had been doing it for so long. I basically brought food to the emotion party of choice—literally! My justification was that I was feeling the emotion AND bringing the food along because I had trained myself that with feeling—any feeling—came intake. This explanation doesn't need to make sense to you. What's important is that it made sense enough to me to realize the mirage I had created and to UNWIND (deprogram) the habit.

I needed to learn to sit with the feeling, without the food. I was already feeling the feeling(s), but the security blanket I had made with the food was indirectly creating many not so good things for me (fat on my body, an addiction to refined sugar, empty feelings that I couldn't connect with because of my blood sugar roller coaster, etc.).

I had to learn to feel my feelings without involving food in the process. I share this in case you are like me. You may be thinking to yourself, "I easily feel all the emotions on this list." Good. Glad you do. But if the answer is no, you have found yourself a trigger that it's time for you to get real with.

List ONE THING (and be specific) that you will start THIS MOMENT to change this. Use your workbook to answer.

Here's another example for you: In her career, my client Sandra often finds herself in conference rooms for full-day meetings. The afternoon "dessert buffet" easily pushes her over the edge. Regardless of techniques attempted, she's unable to stop at one treat. After being cooped up all day long, when the tray arrives at about 2:30 p.m., she's been all but pushed to her limit.

But by recognizing this trigger, she was able to make an essential change: at the 2:30 break, Sandra now fits in a 5-minute breather (regardless of weather, she leaves the session and gets some much-needed fresh air) to change her environment, which gives her a different head space. Also, she packs (from home) her favourite snack for this afternoon window.

Her rule: the tray is for the others (she doesn't tell herself she can't touch the tray, because she knows that would make her want to touch it more!) But if she doesn't start on the tray, she'll have no issue with stopping. A key here, though: her snack needs to be gratifying enough to not be envious of what the others are eating.

Actions

Actions, in the context of triggers, relates to specific things you may do that cause you to eat outside of moderation.

Reflecting on my first days of parenting, in the various book and blogs I read pre-baby, I was reminded to only feed my baby when he was hungry. The experts provided a list of cues and clues on how I'd know that my baby was hungry, versus tired, cranky, or wet.

Pretty straightforward, yes?

So what happens to us as we grow? We stop listening to our basic body cues that we are born with and that our parents learned to watch for and interpret. We edit these cues, make up pretend hunger cues and/or simply eat whenever we choose. These are the actions I'm referring to.

We need to consider several approaches for your success:

1. Using the following template, over the next seven days, record what you eat and what you're doing when you eat it (for example, driving, sitting at the kitchen table with a friend, eating and texting, etc.).

Seriously, take seven days and record this, then come back to the book to keep reading.

	DAY 1	DAY 2	DAY 3	DAY 4	DAY 5	DAY 6	DAY 7
BREAKFAST							
SNACK							
LUNCH							
SNACK							
DINNER							
WATER/OTHER LIQUIDS?							
OTHERS?							
TRIGGER(S)/ FEELING(S)							

Now that you've got a week to review, examine what is triggering you to eat outside of sitting at a table for a meal.

What themes are you seeing in your intake?

_____

_____

_____

I thought it would be helpful if Michelle's clients shared their typical themes for triggered eating. Is this you?

- Rushing to and from work

- Feeding the kids instead of self (and then eating off their plates, followed by eating dinner after kids are in bed, hours later)

- Missing a needed snack

- Eating too much when getting a window of time

- Stress

- Depression

- Boredom

2. Think about a week in your life. Consider how you fill your days and nights. What are you doing with your time outside of work and mealtime? How does that time involve food and how often is it outside your "I must eat because I need energy in my tank to continue?"

Record what you can keep doing, start doing and stop doing to get where you want to be.

_____

_____

_____

3. Picture this: You've had a full day. You haven't stopped since you got up. All you want to do is relax before bed. You decide to _____ (choose from below potential actions or insert your own) and take with you _____(name your food/drink indulgence of choice).

Potential Actions:

- Watch a movie

- Channel surf

- Catch up on e-mail

- Call a friend

- Meditate

- Book club

- Night out with friends

- Post workout snack

- Box Breath

- Play great music

- Other

State two things you're now more aware of because of Action Steps 1-2-3:

_____

_____

_____

"Actions speak louder than words, and are more to be regarded."

Actions may speak louder than words but, for you, do they speak louder than feelings?

Actions or feelings—which are the pivotal point to your trigger eating?

You may think it's your actions (like: I want to lose weight, it feels important to me, yet my actions are weaker than my feelings because regardless of how much I want it, I don't stop myself in the moment of reaching for the snacks brought into my 3 p.m. meeting or the dessert tray the hostess with the most-est pulled out at 8:30 p.m. during book club).

Here's where I'm going to challenge you. You say, "This is important to me, and I want this." Those aren't the feelings I'm talking about. Those feelings are wants—and calling you forth on this, they represent wishful thinking without a plan.

Where you need to get clear, REALLY clear, is specific to this: **what are the feelings that drive you to the action of caving?**

Time to call yourself out on this. You can start your day with intention: "I'm eating healthy today. I am filling my body with nourishment. I yearn for a better body. I strive to eat whole foods."

So far, so good, right? Wrong! You need to have a plan or an intention when the feelings that trigger you into binging arise. Specific examples of these feelings include a reaction or response to:

- Stress (deadlines, crazy expectations, major multi-tasking, etc.)

- Highs to lows (you go go go all day. You get home and the different pace level is like a dip on a roller coaster. It's too much of an extreme so to counterbalance, you use food to bring the energy up a bit)

- Quiet time (you so seldom have time on your own that when you get it you almost feel awkward. Insert food and the feeling goes away)

- A reward mentality (after a long, hard day, you think "I deserve this")

- Self-caring, self-love or development (when a sad feeling hits and whatever comes up for you is something you don't like, aren't used to, or you don't know how to respond, you change the feeling by adding food.

In case we haven't been clear enough, it's time for a frying pan over the head. BANG!

Years of expertise proves that there is a VERY likely chance that your eating triggers are evoked by an emotion or feeling.

Therefore, you—yes, you! —the one wanting to make a lifestyle change—need to live your day like a bystander (for now).

You must acknowledge and note when you are eating and why. Ask yourself what you're feeling. Record the time of day, the food you choose, the feeling you are having. Get real with this. You can't change a habit or trigger if you don't know what the heck you're trying to change.

You have two days. 48 hours. Do this. Create this awareness. Own this change.

DAY 1			DAY 2		
TIME	WHAT I ATE	WHAT I WAS FEELING	TIME	WHAT I ATE	WHAT I WAS FEELING
i.e. 7:45	2 eggs with tomato slice	Hungry, Tired Resisting leaving for work			
i.e. 2:15	Three cookies from staff room	Tired, Bored Energy depletion			

I had the opportunity to participate in a Women's Intensive Retreat run by the amazing, one-of-a-kind Grace Cirocco.

The session deepened my insight on energy and the emotional work I had in front of me.

From the session, I've learned to tap into my emotion by asking myself: "What does my heart say?"

This question can stop me in my tracks. I pause, put my hand to my heart, close my eyes and wait until I have an answer from my heart. With my hand to my heart and my eyes closed, I naturally slow my breathing, which calms and centres me until I have an answer to what my heart is saying.

You know what? My heart's answer is NEVER, "Feed me with food." I listen to what my heart needs, and I make the time to give it that.

Review your notes and the thoughts you have about this chapter so far. In our experience, your triggers are linked to habitual actions, feelings or a mixture of both.

Now that you have awareness of what your triggers are, list the key ones. When we say key, we mean the ones that impact your healthy eating regime more than once a week.

_____

_____

_____

Using this, list the pros and cons of the trigger.

Be specific. REALLY specific.

For example, when I eat while watching television, I turn into a barnyard animal and I will ingest every last scrap from the trough.

TRIGGER	PROS	CONS

If the above cons list isn't clear enough for you to OWN the reasoning behind changing this trigger from your life, what would be? What is going to make you deprogram this trigger once and for all?

ANSWER THIS.

_____

_____

_____

Chapter 6: (Part 1) Keys to G

- You're reading this book to make different choices for your life.

- You are reading this book because it is time to take care of you. To do for yourself what no else can do for you.

- You are reading this book because you deserve to have your life, all of it.

- Triggers suck. They are habits worth changing. Make them anything more than that and they win your life. Make them only habits and POOF! You win the power to do with them what you wish.

Part 2 - The Trigger Replacement Plan

First, take a deep breath. A good, full-diaphragm, big exhale on the way out, cleansing deep breath.

Part 1 of Triggers was hardcore. The realness of where you went for yourself (a.k.a. The Emotional Trigger Dig) is deserved and required for your personal success. Now that you have that knowledge, let's use it for your benefit and success.

The trigger replacement plan consists of some self-love, present moment awareness and clarity of your values/what you want to lead with.

Self-love. Yes, it sounds a little hippie-ish… and maybe that's why I like it! Considering the emotions you uncovered above, it's time to refill your well.

So what does self-love mean?

To me, it's nourishing your soul. It's about loving yourself fully first, so that you can fully love others by understanding and respecting your own well-being and creating your own happiness.

Key words for me in this definition:

- Nourishing your soul

- Respecting your own well-being

- Creating your own happiness

- Loving yourself fully

Choosing any of the four components within the self-love definition will give you a similar answer. Select which one fits best for you and record it, then describe it.

Self-love

_____ means to me:

_____

_____

_____

Having this fully would feel like:

_____

_____

_____

Which would allow me to:

_____

_____

_____

We need to learn to be kind to ourselves, nourishing ourselves and satisfying with different emotional desires.

Why? Because nourishing this need with food and/or binging is not working. And in some cases this fix may even be killing you slowly.

Here's a sample of what this exercise, completed, might look like:

Nourishing My Soul

This is what nourishing my soul means to me:

Being aware of my feelings (positive and negative), and acknowledging them for myself by naming them and feeling their impact on me.

Breathing. Taking time in my day to literally connect to my BEing. Centering myself to what's important to me, so I keep that the focus, versus running mindlessly through my day.

Laughing at myself. As I continue to let go of my preconceived notion of what others think I should be, or who I think I should be, I will learn to giggle as I misstep.

Spending time outside. It keeps me grounded!

Did I mention breathing? Be aware of the crazy tempo I'm used to, and be aware of what I lose when I don't take a moment to breathe.

Having this fully would feel:

- Easy

- Like a movie with a good ending!

- Freeing

- In control

Which would allow me to:

- BE me—all of me.

Wow… yep, now I get it. I need to own this!

In the example above, the client realized the importance of what she needed to do and how it fit with the life value she admired.

Now, it comes down to connecting the what and the value(s) you acknowledged, and from that, create the how. Reviewing the notes in your self-love exercise, how will you apply this, to create this habit?

Please note: this is not a Nice To-Do task, but a Must-Do, if you want to be successful.

The practice starts today—and continues every day.

Starting today I will: (be as specific as possible)

_____

_____

_____

You can find this exercise in the workbook!

=>> http://bonus.weightlossgspot.com

Chapter 6: (Part 2) Keys to G

- Trigger is a buzzword these days. Be cognizant of the ease of labeling a trigger and using it as an excuse versus what it really is—an explanation of what has caused you (in the past) to do something. That's it. Time to change it. Your life, your choices.

- My choice is to be trigger-free!

7

ENJOY THE RIDE

Michelle here… Are you ready to officially kick off your new food plan? Here we go.

Close your eyes. Sit back and relax—and picture your ideal self. What do you look like?

What are you wearing?

How do you feel?

What is your mood?

I know you have imagined this ideal self a thousand times, if not a million. This ideal self (remember, the self you wrote about) is now ready to take that next step towards looking, feeling and being EXACTLY what you want.

_____

_____

_____

You can find this exercise in the workbook!

=>> http://bonus.weightlossgspot.com

Deep down inside, you know what you want. The great news is that maybe, without recognizing it, you've already worked through—and maybe even completed—some of the hardest parts of this journey!

First, you decided that your status quo wasn't good enough. Awesome!

Many people simply get stuck in their own rut, never really realizing that there's more out there, whatever their more is.

Second, you took action by purchasing this book.

This stage of discovery is major. Why not find out what options are out there for you, right?

Third, you've put pen to paper in the form of goal-setting and self-discovery, and you're ready now to take action on your dreams.

I've found that the action step is often the hardest part. Many of us fail to start because we are worried it won't be seamless and that we might fail before we even start. The very fact you've started speaks volumes. It's true this journey might not have been easy so far, but sometimes the things in life that are most worthwhile are also the hardest.

There comes a time in each of our lives when finally, all the thinking, planning, hoping, dreaming and goal-setting is over. It's GO time—and I think you're ready!

You've taken all the right steps forward and now are you're here. Welcome!

Let's do this together. We'll be here for you every step of the way.

The 3-G Pillar Program

The 3-G Pillar Program was designed with weight loss ease in mind, meaning the concepts are simple to follow and then maintain. If you abide by the parameters set here, weight loss is typically inevitable.

One of the first questions I encounter when designing a program for someone is, "How much will I lose and how quickly?"

My response is always the same:

1. It took you _____ many years to get where you are now, so if your goal is to lose 20 to 100 pounds, than you need to expect that this will take some time. Make peace with this.

2. Age, gender, activity level, stress, pre-existing health conditions (including use of medication), sleep patterns, hormonal imbalance created partially by extra body fat and more, all play a role—so it's difficult to exactly predict these kind of things.

> *Nancy here: WHOA, G readers! This is about the journey. You've already completed your vision board. Now, focus on the journey to get there, versus how much, how fast.*
>
> *BREATHE. Be kind to yourself. When you rush, there's no orgasm. You know what I'm talking about, ladies! Enjoy the ride versus looking to the prize!*

Even so, if you follow through with the program, typically you can expect to lose about 1 to 2 lb. per week, on average. Know that there will be some weeks that you lose nothing and others when you might lose more, even though you're doing the same things.

I often hear moans and groans when I explain that one pound per week is the average loss for women (men, you can expect a bit more).

Instead of focusing on how little one pound per week might seem, focus on this:

One pound is equivalent to a brick of butter. Yes, you read that right. Go pick up a brick of butter right now. Do it! Feel how big and heavy that brick is? Losing one whole brick of butter off your body each week is significant. Trust me.

> *Nancy here: Interesting that Michelle and I both talk weight in terms of butter. Dare you to unwrap the butter Michelle just told you to pick up. Dare you to smoosh and squeeze the butter between your fingers. Kinda looks like fat, yes? Imagine 1 or 2 of those bricks coming off your body every week. That's a HUGE win.*

3. One of the biggest misconceptions out there is that weight loss is just about calories in versus calories out.

In actuality, you need to factor in your age, lifestyle, gastrointestinal health, activity level (or lack of), stress, medical conditions (medications), hormonal imbalance, sleep and genetics. If you are at all struggling through the weight loss process, ensure you are considering the other factors that affect your ability to drop the weight as well.

How Stress Can Affect Weight Loss

I met Suzanne two years ago when she came to me in hopes of losing 15 to 20 pounds. Suzanne is, and was always, an active individual.

She trained for and ran marathons, worked out several times a week with her personal trainer and practiced yoga regularly. Her diet wasn't perfect but with some small changes, I figured we would have her down in no time.

Much to my surprise, a month and a half later, we were still stuck at the same weight. By this time, it was clear we were dealing with something more than just what she was eating and expending.

Suzanne led a hectic life, both career-wise and personally, so I decided to take another route with her and concentrate on reducing her stress and anxiety.

The effects that stress and anxiety can have on the body can slow down or prevent people from losing body fat. When you're stressed or anxious, a hormone called cortisol is released into your system. One of the main functions of cortisol is to tell your body to store fat, a response that goes back to our days as hunters and gatherers.

The body is smart—in times of drought or famine, fat is stored and calories conserved as a survival mechanism. In long ago times, cortisol release was helpful in keeping people alive. Fast forward to today and our cortisol release is being triggered by traffic jams, deadlines and chaos at home.

The changes Suzanne had to make were significant, if she were to see any results. She had to completely reset the way her body perceived the environment around her. We introduced herbal support and other forms of stress management techniques to help her cope better (see Chapter 10 for more details).

Sure enough, 2 to 3 months later, after some soul searching and lifestyle adjustments, Suzanne came in for her appointment—and she had dropped six pounds! What a great start for her weight loss journey.

Fact is, there are no "for sures" when it comes to weight loss, but here are Nancy's top three tips to keep you motivated:

- *Clear your intention. Every morning, I give myself a couple of extra minutes to lie in bed and connect with my day. This includes me considering how I want to show up, how I want to handle myself with food and how I will say yes to choosing my G-Spot. Be clear. Be specific. Be real.*

- *Be with the change. What does this mean? Every day, pre- or post-shower, I stand in front of the mirror naked (women over the age of ____, you are welcome to stand with your hands above your head. I sometimes do this to remind my breasts to go back where they came from). Then, OUT LOUD, I acknowledge five things I like that I see based on the efforts I'm making.*

- *Get others involved. Share your goals with others and have them on your team. Explain what this means to you and how you'll need their help, support, encouragement and love. Have them sprinkle these gifts at random with you, and be clear how often you need it. Know how to ask for it easily.*

3:2:1 Go!

Okay, folks, this is it! This is the real deal. This is what you've been working toward. It's finally GO TIME!

The actual guts of this weight loss program are built around three simple steps:

Pillar 1 is our Toss the Worn-Out Panties stage. This means taking away those so-called "foods" that only serve to hinder your efforts.

Pillar 2 is our Change Room Try-Outs stage. Like speed dating, this is your opportunity to test the waters, so to speak. Here you will begin to understand your new lifestyle habits and the rules you'll live by if you want to lose weight and keep it off!

Pillar 3 is the "I've Got This" stage, where you're walked through those foods you should be consuming on a daily basis to facilitate healthy fat loss. That's it! It's that simple.

Pillar 1: Toss The Worn-Out Panties!

This particular phase of the program is aimed at balancing your blood sugar and hormonal systems. Why is this important? Very simply, when blood sugars are balanced, hormones are more likely to be balanced and weight loss is much easier.

> *Nancy here: It's like this. You date a guy for a while. You try and try and try but finally, you get it that he's not The One. You break it off with him. This is like that phase. The prep-yourself to get back-in-the-game phase. The game is Find My Weight Loss G-Spot.*

Here's why.

Sugar and Fat: The Connection

"Insulin plays a significant role in sugar usage and fat storage. Normally, the carbohydrates you eat get converted to sugar. As sugar levels rise, insulin is secreted by the pancreas to transport sugar into the cells to be used as fuel (energy). During optimal conditions, insulin production is limited to the amount needed to stimulate the metabolism of the ingested carbohydrate (sugars).

However, the excessive consumption of carbohydrates can throw off this delicate and precise dynamic between insulin and blood sugar and lead to too much insulin production."

As the cycle continues (more and more insulin being secreted) your body becomes accustomed to these levels and therefore requires more insulin to do its original job.

"As insulin gets secreted in higher and higher dosage, it sweeps sugar out of the blood and into the cells, causing blood sugar levels to drop. This drop in blood sugar levels triggers a craving for more sugar. If you succumb to this craving, you stimulate more insulin secretion and another drop in blood sugar, which in turn provokes more sugar cravings, sugar consumption, and ultimately another rise in insulin secretion, and so on."

When your blood sugars are low from too much insulin secretion (due to the consumption of too much sugars and carbohydrates), it is at this time your body feels fatigued (generally before and after lunch).

Unless stopped, this pattern of carbohydrate/sugar ingestion, subsequent energy lows, followed by cravings and again and the ultimate ingestion of these foods will wreak havoc on the body (causing fat accumulation), and mind.

Simply put, Pillar 1 emphasizes the removal of the top three major weight loss offenders, the "foods" that hinder, slow or even bring weight loss to a grinding halt.

These are:

1. White flours (in particular, wheat)

2. Obvious processed sugars

3. Hidden sources of sugar

Now, hear me out, I totally understand you're thinking, "Duh, I know this already, dammit, and it hasn't helped me at all." I truly believe, though, that I need to drive this point home.

These are, in fact, the foods that give most people trouble. If you're looking for a magic fix, it isn't out there. Getting a grip on the point above, however, will get you to you to Your Weight Loss G-Spot.

Here are some more facts that help prove my point.

The concept that these "foods" above are essentially useless, devoid of any nutritional value, isn't new or radical thinking. The prevalence of gluten and wheat sensitivities has become mainstream and who, in this day and age, hasn't heard that sugar is the root of all evil?

NO ONE! Then why, despite the warnings, do people still struggle with this temptation?

First and foremost, I think the media is doing a great job of sending us mixed messages. On one hand, the experts are telling us that processed white flours and sugars are junk; that they create inflammation in the body, a major ingredient for chronic disease.

On the other hand, we are lured by fancy marketing and our desire for convenience into consuming these foods.

Cravings and chemical imbalances are key reasons why many simply cannot follow through easily with the elimination of these foods. When these items are consumed they cause us to temporarily feel really good… euphoric, actually.

Refined white flours and sugars help with the absorption of an amino acid called tryptophan (yes, the same amino acid that makes us feel sleepy and content after we eat a big turkey dinner). Then, this triggers serotonin to be secreted (our "happy" chemical).

This chemical reaction makes us feel super content in that moment so why would we not want whatever food created this drug-like effect?

Simultaneously, another hormone called insulin is released and the result of this is a blood sugar drop. What does this mean? Very simply, whatever you are eating will be associated with happiness. Remember this! This is, in essence, a false high.

At the same time, your blood sugars are dropping and your body naturally wants to counteract this uncomfortable development by stimulating you to unconsciously to eat something with sugar to bring your blood sugars back up and create that happy feeling all over again. If you need to, refer back to that cookie example from Chapter 4.

Also worth noting: I strongly believe many people are simply not sure how to go about implementing change. Whether it's because they don't have the education, a good support system or simply because it feels too hard, change is tough and is often closely tied to the way we view the world. Let's do something about that!

Let this book serve as the starting point to your education on healthy foods and lifestyle. You don't need to be an expert to make good changes.

A good support system is important. If you don't have one right from the beginning, focus on positive changes for yourself. You'll find people often follow suit.

Starting now, it's all about your attitude. You can choose to feel sorry for yourself because you feel "restricted" or you can dive into what you know will be a positive new shift in the way you lead your life. Embrace change!

I promise that once you get into the swing of things and notice all the positive changes, you won't want to go back to the way it used to be. Clients always tell me that this new way of life feels normal once they get into the swing of things.

My story: *A few years ago it was suggested to me that I consider a wheat-free/gluten-free lifestyle. I was suffering from some pretty major gastrointestinal issues, a discomfort that would plague me the better part of the day (gas, bloating—all the gross stuff!)*

As a nutritionist, I embraced this change… or I thought I did. As the months wore on, dinners out, parties and family gatherings proved to be quite difficult. It wasn't for the lack of wheat- and gluten-free options, but more to do with my frame of mind about this new lifestyle. Foods that I used to order or eat without much thought were now off limits.

I found that I was getting upset and feeling sorry for myself because of this. It wasn't fair that everyone else around me got to have whatever they wanted and I couldn't! I went to Jamaica later that year and used it as an excuse to fall off the wagon.

At the beginning of 2013, my goal was to resume my wheat- free and gluten-free lifestyle… this time with a new attitude. Instead of fighting it and feeling sorry for myself, I decided to make peace with it.

At the end of the day, this is a choice I've made. I've decided on my own to live my life this way; therefore, I also refuse to get upset about it.

Don't get me wrong, sometimes I am bummed I can't have a hunk of white Italian bread, but eventually I get over it by remembering the bigger picture and how I felt before my lifestyle transition… then I find something I can have and move on. Remember, it's all about choices.

Now, going back to our top three offenders.

The reason I choose to dedicate two categories out of three to sugars is this: it's an area that still seems to elude many clients in my private practice. Most of us know when we are consuming obvious sources of sugar (in our coffee, candy and desserts). However, it's the hidden sources of sugar that can be just as troublesome to losing weight, if not more, simply because we are unaware of their presence. Examples like juices, flavoured yogurts, many grain products and granola cereals usually have a mountain of sugar in them and simply removing these from your day-to-day diet can sometimes make all the difference.

Here is a list of common household "foods" that contain obvious, hidden and unnecessary (to finding Your Weight Loss G-spot) forms of sugar.

OBVIOUS SUGARY "FOOD" EXAMPLES	NOT SO OBVIOUS SUGARY "FOOD" EXAMPLES	NOTES
	Canned fruit (or other canned vegetables)	This is referring to the products with sugar water for preservation
	Baked beans	Sugar is added for sweetness
	Instant oatmeal	Often contains white sugar and artificial sweeteners
Cookies		
Pastries like muffins and croissants		
Candy and chocolate		
Pop		
	Sports drinks like Gatorade	Many have artificial colours and flavours too
Alcohol		
	Bottled sauces likes teriyaki and sweet and sour	Why did you think they are so yummy? That's right, chalk full of sugar!
	Frozen, ready-made meals	
Ice cream		
Jello and puddings (even the sugar-free varieties)		
	Fresh or concentrated juices	You end up consuming more than just one serving of fruit when you drink juice; therefore you consume more sugar than intended
	Flavoured yogurts	In addition to the natural sugars in the fruit, the fruit bottom is often also loaded with extra sugars
Jams, jellies and syrups		
Beer		
	Flavoured milks and alternative milks like (soy, coconut, rice and almond)	Choose natural and unsweetened options
	Many protein powders and bars	Lots of sugar makes them more palatable

Recap: How's that for a realization of the "sugar world" you've been living in? Which four food items are tripping you up most with sugar ingestion AND what will you do differently from this moment on?

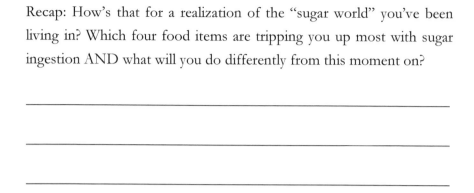

White grains (flours) are proving to be as problematic as the sugars. Because of their convenience, additives and newfound hybrid genetic makeup, thanks to agri-business, white flours (wheat) specifically, and other gluten containing grains are popping up as the culprit to not only weight issues but many common health concerns. According to author William Davis of the popular book *Wheat Belly*, "eliminating wheat from our diets can prevent fat storage, shrink unsightly bulges, and reverse a myriad of health problems".

Although wheat is the most popular, and therefore, I'd argue the biggest, concern, I could argue that all grains (corn, rice, oats, spelt, rye, etc.) can all be problematic for those trying to lose weight (if not eaten in moderation).

The thought of going wheat- or grain-free permanently for many is unthinkable—and I agree this can be unnecessary most of the time. What is necessary, though, is reducing these hard-to-digest, inflammation-triggering, craving-rousing, just-gotta-have-them foods.

Here is a short list of common grain-based products (not limited to just wheat-based products) that many people consume daily, if not several times a day.

Reducing—not eliminating—these will not only force you into making different and arguably better choices, but will also… and trust me on this… help you lose weight.

- White breads

- Crackers, white pasta

- Oatmeal and oat products like granola bars

- White rice and rice based products

- Corn and corn based products like tortillas

Initially, removing some of the grain products from your day-to-day diet will be a challenge.

Knowing this up front, embrace the change! That's why you're here, for change.

The below list of replacement foods will be helpful with the transition process.

If you end up feeling slightly sluggish or some fatigue sets in, know this is most likely temporary because we have removed some simple carbohydrates (also known as sugar!) from your diet.

Within a week (maximum two weeks), you will feel like yourself again, but the 2.0, happier, more energized version!

Keep reading for a list of common symptoms you can experience when changing your diet and lifestyle.

IF YOU MISS:	TRY THIS:
BREAD	Cloud Bread – you will find this as well as other great recipes and free resources at http://bonus.weightlossgspot.com
PASTA	Baked spaghetti squash or pasta made from beans and lentil (check out this brand: Explore Asian: Authentic Cuisine and Tolerant Foods lentil pasta)
RICE	Revamped Rice Recipe – you will find this as well as other great recipes and free resources at http://bonus.weightlossgspot.com

In order to get the most out of this change, Pillar 1 will last one week.

In this time frame, you'll be eliminating many of the "foods" that have led you to this point.

These were the "foods" that made you feel sluggish, unwell, interrupted your sleep, created bloating and that extra tire-ring around your belly!

In Chapter 5, we spent some time "boxing it," cleaning out the kitchen/pantry and tossing those "foods" that lead you astray. Celebrate that you have done this and stayed away from the majority of these G-Spot-busters!

G Is For Go

For the next seven days, for simplicity, you're going to commit yourself to the meals provided below.

Why, you ask? This will be the first step in getting you back in control of your food-based decisions! I've just made it really simple for you.

My advice for starting:

- Set yourself up for success. The kitchen must be free of those trigger foods, with fresh, healthy options available and ready to go.

- Plan your meals ahead of time. My most successful clients are those who make a plan for the week, stock their kitchen accordingly and follow through with this plan—which leads to my third piece of advice.

- Prep! Prep, prep and prep some more. Having healthy options available will ensure you have something to grab when hunger or a craving strikes. Remember, if I got to my next meal and nothing healthy was available, I'd grab the Doritos, too!

Tip: Plan ahead and use the shopping list created for you in the Resources and References section at the end of the book.

Please pick one option from each meal category daily for 7 days:

Breakfast:

1. 2-3 eggs, any style, with 1 slice of sprouted grain bread (Ezekiel or Stonemill) or a gluten-free option (make sure it's not white bread).

2. Smoothie made from preapproved protein powders (see list in Chapter 4), blended with water or unsweetened almond, rice, hemp, coconut or soy milk or regular cow's milk. Optional ingredients include: ½ cup berries, baby spinach, ground flax seeds, pure vanilla extract, cinnamon, 1 tsp. coconut oil.

3. 1 cup cottage cheese or plain Greek yogurt (0% or 2% is fine). Optional ingredients: cinnamon, pure vanilla extract, ½ cup fruit, 3 tbsp. raw nuts or seeds, ¼ cup uncooked plain oatmeal

WANT MORE DELICIOUS, FREE RECIPES?

Get access to all of your free bonus resources at
http://bonus.weightlossgspot.com/

Lunch:

1. Tuna Salad: (canned or fresh) served over large green salad (and any other vegetables) with olive oil and lemon dressing (1 tbsp. each), topped with cracked pepper and sea salt. Optional ingredients: ¼ avocado, mustard, 1 tsp. mayonnaise.

2. Inspired Greek Chicken Salad: Chicken breast served over roughly chopped bell peppers, red onion and any other vegetables and ½ cup chickpeas (or any bean of your choice). Dressing: 1 tbsp. olive oil, splash of red wine vinegar and a pinch of each dried oregano and basil, sea salt and pepper. Optional ingredients: 8 olives, 2 oz goat or feta cheese, ½ whole wheat or gluten free pita (remember no white pitas)

   * feel free to substitute with 3 tbsp. hemp seeds instead of chicken

3. Open-Faced Egg Salad Sandwich: 2 hardboiled eggs served in ½ a whole wheat or gluten-free pita or served over 1 slice sprouted grain or gluten-free bread. Pair this with some veggies and ¼ cup hummus dip (homemade or purchased). Optional ingredients: 1 tsp. mayo, ¼ avocado, mustard, sea salt, pepper.

4. Leftovers from dinners

Dinner:

1. BBQ or baked chicken, fish or lean beef with sweet potato and side veggie of your choice

2. Chicken or Turkey Chili with side of any 2 green veggies.

3. Baked Chicken Casserole over mashed "potato" aka cauli-smash

4. One Pot Turkey Cabbage Slaw

*make double portions so you have left overs for the next day

Dinner Recipes

BBQ or baked chicken, fish or lean beef with Sweet Potato

Season any herbs, spices, sea salt and pepper and serve with any green vegetable and sweet potato oven wedges.

Instructions for wedges: 1 small sweet potato cut into wedges. Brushed with olive oil and sprinkled with sea salt, pepper and paprika. Preheat over to 400F. Turn over after 20 minutes and leave in oven for another 15-20 minutes until soft and slightly browned.

Turkey/Chicken Chili

Ingredients:

- 1 lbs minced turkey or1 lbs skinless chicken breast, cubed

- 1 sweet onion (chopped)

- 3 tbsp. grape seed or olive oil

- 1 can lentils (rinsed)

- 1 can black beans (rinsed)

- 1 20 oz canned or fresh diced tomatoes

- Pinch cayenne pepper

- 1 tsp. cumin

- 1tsp. garlic powder

- ½ tsp. dried oregano

- 1 tsp. sea salt

- ½ tsp. ground pepper

Directions:

Sautee onions and meat until browned (this gives them more flavour).

Transfer all of the ingredients to slow cooker or large stove-top pot.

Stir in remaining ingredients.

Cover and cook over low heat for 3-5 hours.

Enjoy!

Makes 4 servings

Lemon Baked Chicken and Bean Casserole

Ingredients:

- 1 yukon gold potato or purple potato thinly sliced (use a mandolin if you have one)

- ½ tsp. sea salt

- 2 medium sized carrots (peeled)

- ½ tsp. smoked paprika

- 1 tbsp. garlic powder

- 2 tsp. olive oil

- 1 can navy or black beans (rinsed and drained)

- 4 chicken legs

- 1 lemon sliced into rounds

- 4 garlic cloves (minced)

Directions:

Preheat oven to 400F

Place whole carrots and potato in the bottom of a baking dish. Sprinkle with ¼ tsp. sea salt, garlic powder and cloves and paprika. Drizzle 1 tsp. olive oil over mixture.

Now top with beans.

On the beans, lay the slices from one lemon.

Season chicken legs both sides with remaining olive oil, sea salt and paprika and place over lemons.

Season dish with pepper. Roast for 1 to 1.5 hours or until chicken is golden brown. Serve with a spinach salad and/or a smashed "potato".

Makes 2 servings

Cauli-smash

Ingredients:

- 1 head of cauliflower rinsed and cut into florets

- 1-2 clove garlic

- 1tbsp. olive oil

- 1tsp. parmesan cheese

- sea salt and pepper to taste

Directions:

Place cauliflower and garlic in pot and boil until tender (1 inch of water is enough).

Once cooked pour out excess water (careful not to spill out the garlic).

Add 1 tbsp. olive oil and use a food processor or immersion hand blender to whip the cauliflower and garlic into a mash.

Add salt, parmesan and pepper for flavor.

One-Pot Turkey Cabbage Slaw

Ingredients:

- 1 pound ground turkey (organic where possible)
- ¼ tsp. sea salt
- ¼ tsp. black pepper
- ½ tsp. onion powder
- ½ tsp. garlic powder
- 1-2 pounds of cabbage or 1 bag of coleslaw
- 1 tsp. garlic, minced
- 2 tbsp. sesame oil
- 2 tbsp. low sodium soy sauce or tamari sauce

- 2 tbsp. Frank's hot sauce

- 2 tsp. apple cider vinegar

- 1 tsp. raw honey or agave

- ½ tsp. red pepper, crushed (optional)

Directions:

In a pan, add the beef, salt, pepper, garlic powder, and onion powder.

Let this finish on the stove with a lid on (it will only take a minute).

While this is cooking, chop up the cabbage. Make sure you shred it very thin. An optional choice is to use an already prepared shredded coleslaw mix.

Scoop out the ground beef into a medium sized bowl. Leave as much oil as possible in the pan.

To the pan, add minced garlic, sesame oil, and the shredded cabbage. Let that cook. It's done when you can see it getting brown on the bottom.

Add soy sauce, hot sauce, apple cider vinegar, and honey or agave to cabbage. Give it a stir.

Now, add the ground beef back into the frying pan.

Optional: add crushed red pepper to the mix.

Enjoy!

Makes 6 Servings

(Recipe adapted from Atkins Diet)

Snacks:

(pick two or three options per day, to be eaten between main meals)

1. 1 apple and 1 tbsp. nut butter

2. Cucumber and broccoli (or any veggie) dipped in ¼ cup homemade ranch dip (add ½ tsp. dried dill, a pinch of sea salt and pepper, ½ clove minced garlic clove, 1 tbsp. parmesan cheese, 2 tbsp. olive oil to 1/4 cup plain Greek yogurt.

3. 8 olives and carrots dipped in hummus (bought or made)

4. 12 almonds and ½ cup berries

5. Fresh tomatoes drizzled with olive oil. Add a pinch of sea salt and pepper and fresh basil and 1 Laughing Cow or BabyBel or 1 oz mozzarella cheese.

6. ½ cup plain yogurt, cottage cheese or ricotta with ½ cup berries, with side of veggies

Cravings

A craving, as defined by Webster.com, is: "an intense, urgent, or abnormal desire or longing."

This is what I tell all my clients when it comes to these nasty want-to-eat-everything-and-anything-I-can-find-to-satisfy-this craving feeling.

Please know cravings will subside a few days after sugars and white grains (flours) have been eliminated from your diet.

We know this phase can sometimes be tough, so we encourage the following if you are struggling with cravings:

- Chew gum

- Brush your teeth

- Drink herbal tea

- Sleep

- Take a warm bath or shower

- Get distracted: read, take a walk, find a hobby, talk to a friend

- Dance!

- Stopping yourself in that moment and ask, "Is this really hunger?" If the answer is "NO," identify what you're really feeling (tired, for example) and figure out what you need to do instead of eat to address that feeling!

- Find your G-Spot!

Please also know this—a craving will not kill you!

Despite what you might be thinking in the throes of an urge, know you will not perish if you do not fulfill the craving. Logically, we know this to be true, but I've heard some stories about what lengths people will go to quiet the cravings.

Advice and Strategies From My Clients:

Let's get right to the source and find out thoughts and strategies my clients find helpful when a craving strikes:

"I think if I didn't have a dessert planned for Sunday nights, I would end up craving sweets more often. Instead, I research my recipes and ensure that the dessert is a smaller portion size than before and is delicious and consistent with the clean eating style I'm now enjoying." ~Sarah

"Prevent the cravings! I never let myself get hungry. Eat a healthy fat between meals, like Greek yogurt, 12 almonds or hummus and veggies." ~Darcy

"I often have a craving because I can see the food or know it is in the house. To prevent the craving, try to not have "bad foods" in the house." ~Darcy

"At the end of the day, it's a decision. You choose either path. If you say "yes" to a craving, make peace with it and skip the guilt." ~Diane

"A tough, but effective, strategy has been to keep a food journal. When this commitment is made, it stops you from consuming all those chips, chocolate, etc. Who wants to honestly record those items? When I've followed the food plan, made healthy choices, am neither full nor hungry, it becomes quite easy to divert myself during those moments when temptation arises. The feeling of success is sweet indeed!" ~Erika

"It's important to forgive yourself and just get going again. No one criticizes me the way that I can, so it's taken some work to learn that's it's okay, to just stop beating up on myself, redirect my focus and to simply continue with the journey. Smile! You can do this!" ~Erika

"Become aware of patterns and triggers and identify alternative activities that are enjoyable. For me, having wine with dinner often triggers a craving for salt.

Replacing the wine with sparkling water, flavoured water with lemon or lime, or sipping a glass of Kombucha (a recent discovery), are obvious alternatives. Another trigger has been watching TV in the evening and associating yummy snacks with enjoying a show. It's been helpful to change the patterns." ~Erika

"I paint my nails!" ~Dianne

"Work on a craft, like knitting or painting—anything that will keep your hands busy."~Dianne

"When a craving hits, I find it best to just give in—but with a substitute for a cleaner version. Honestly, these days I prefer the cleaner version anyhow, and the best part is that there is no guilt afterwards." ~Victoria

"There have been nights when I was having a really tough time with a craving (chocolate was hard to give up in the early stages). Having my husband there to support me and say, "You can do this!" helped. We'll now go upstairs at 10 p.m. and watch TV in bed instead of being on the main floor, where the kitchen—and temptations lurk." ~Liz

Please note:

Changes in hunger: Feeling hungry or very full the first week (or two weeks) is very common. Often this is just a sign that the body is adjusting to the changes in food quantity and quality. Work through it! If you are feeling really full than consider decreasing your portion sizes at each meal marginally, but stick with the meal and snack program.

If you're hungry, make sure you're drinking lots of water. This can help keep you feeling full. Consider vegetables "free" as well, so have as many of these as you want.

Bowel movements: Could become looser or more constipated.

If you are constipated, consider these solutions:

- Drink more water (add fresh lemon)

- Eat more green veggies

- Add 1 tbsp. flax or chia seeds to a smoothie or salad daily

- If your bowel movements are loose, know this is probably temporary due to increased fibre, water or just a little stress with the change in your diet and lifestyle. This should correct itself fairly quickly.If this persists for more than a week please back off on some of your raw veggies (lightly cook instead), get extra sleep, watch your stress levels, drink lots of water and consider checking in with your GP.

Fatigue: Often the reduction in simple sugars will results in some fatigue for a week or two. This, too, shall pass!

Consider the following tips for getting through this time:

- Get more sleep! Set a bedtime for yourself. Set a timer to alert you to stick to this bedtime.

- Water will help flush the system and hydrate your brain.

- Reduce stress during this time. Stress is very tiring to the body (see Chapter 10 for strategies).

- Get enough lean proteins—eggs, poultry and plant-based proteins like hemp and clean protein powders.

- Move your body! Even light walking can help perk you up.

Cravings: are not uncommon in the first few weeks. When you reduce or eliminate certain foods that your body is used to, cravings can occur. They can be frustrating to work through, but after avoiding your biggest temptations for 4 to 7 days (on average), that craving will most likely disappear.

Weight gain: Some people do gain weight the first week. This happens when your body is adjusting to a difference in calories. Typically, it takes one week for this to correct itself and you should start losing-so don't panic!

Remember that this is the fresh start you have been imagining and dreaming about! It starts today!

Pillar 1 is the most difficult. Once you complete it, you'll not only feel better but you'll enter Pillar 2 with a greater sense of control and motivation!

It's time. Start your seven days. Live your seven days to the best of your ability!

GO!

Pillar 2: Change Room Try-Outs

The following simple concepts will help you with decisions surrounding when and what to eat and drink. Following the week of Pillar 1, Pillar 2 concepts will coincide with the foods outlined in Pillar 3.

The goal here is to combine the concepts of Pillar 2 with the foods from Pillar 3. You will follow these two Pillars until you have reached your weight loss goal.

I'll say this again so it's really clear. Pillar 2 and 3 happen simultaneously and will take you the distance. They are the 'meat and potatoes' of your weight loss food program. Now go get'em tiger!

Pillar 2 Concepts, Guidelines, Rules… call them whatever you want!

1. Please have breakfast, lunch, afternoon snack and dinner daily. Aim to eat a small meal or snack approximately every three hours. If you would like to have a morning snack (and I highly recommend that you do), please enjoy! The purpose of this is to ensure your metabolic rate stays active and constantly burning calories. In addition, consuming healthy, fresh, protein-rich foods through the day will keep your blood sugar stabilized, preventing that oh-so-uncomfortable energy dip.

2. Please consume all the foods (no more and no less!) on the G-Spot Friendly Foods list (below) each day. Please do not eat more than one protein per meal; spread these out over your day. Doing this will ensure you are consuming enough macro and micronutrients to support healthy fat loss.

3. Ideally, dinner should be eaten before 7:30 p.m. Avoid eating after 7:30 p.m. anything other than foods from the "free" list. The reason for this is two-fold. One, calories that most of us crave in the evenings are high-carbohydrate, junky foods that most likely will not get burned off in the later hours of the day. Secondly, these hard-to-digest foods disrupt the detoxification that happens during the night and replaces it with digestion—one sure way to become toxic and not sleep well!

4. Please have eight cups of fresh water per day. In addition to this, you may have 1-2 coffees or black teas per day.

You may add 1 tsp. of honey, agave or stevia to this if you currently use sugar. You may also use cow's milk or unsweetened coconut, rice, cashew, almond, hemp or soy milks. No cream, please.

Here's a list of other G-Spot Friendly Beverages:

- Water (duh!)

- Herbal tea (hot and cold)

- Homemade smoothies made with fresh fruit, water, veggies, healthy fats and unsweetened milks

- Soda water with fresh lemon or lime (1-2 per day—the rest should be still water)

5. Treats are to be limited to three servings per week in Pillar 2. For the sake of simplicity, treats are anything not found on your G-Spot Foods list and are 150 calories or less each.

Here are some examples of treats:

- A 4oz glass of wine (red is preferred)

- 1 bottle of beer

- 1 oz spirit mixed with water, tonic, soda, diluted juice

- 2-3 squares of 85% and above dark chocolate. My favourite is the Endangered Species brand

- 100-150 calories of chips, candy

- A small slice of cake or pie (about as thick as your index and middle finger combined)

> **Tip:** Remember the "pick your poison" strategy from before? Choose only those treats you really love and don't waste your treat on those "foods" that you don't really care for.

We're really moving along!

Now that you have the parameters for how and when to eat, Pillar 3 explains what and how much.

Pillar 3: I've Got This

The following chart represents the number of servings of each food group you need to consume each day in order to healthfully lose body fat.

This might be more or less food than you are used to having. If this is the case, I recommend reminding yourself of all the positive experiences you'll reap by changing your diet.

You will find below a sample meal plan to start with. You can use this or have more flexibility by creating your own. It's your choice.

The serving suggestions below are based upon the average woman. If your weight on the scale is over 150 lb., please consume four proteins per day instead of three. If three servings isn't enough and you are 150 lbs. or less, go ahead and have four servings of protein too.

1 serving = ½ cup unless otherwise marked.

3 SERVINGS/DAY	2 SERVINGS/DAY	1 SERVING/DAY
PROTEIN: 1 SERVING=4-5 OZ	FRUIT:	GRAINS:
Poultry: chicken, turkey, pheasant, quail, duck, goose, hen Game: bison, venison, elk Lean beef: flank, hamburger Pork (loin, chops) Eggs Lamb Fish: salmon, cod, bass, haddock, halibut, perch, herring, tilapia, trout mackerel, pike, sardines, tuna Shellfish: shrimp, oysters, scallops, mussels, crab, lobster Tofu Tempeh Soy burgers Cottage cheese (¾ cup, 0%) Plain Greek yogurt (¾ cup, 0%) Ricotta cheese (½ cup, 0%) Protein powder (from list on page 15 in Chapter 5) Protein bars (Simply bar or Quest bar [sucralose-free])	Apple (1) Pear (1) Peach (1) Cherries Plum (1) Cantaloupe Berries: raspberries, blueberries, blackberries, strawberries Banana (½) Watermelon Kiwi (2) Mango (½) Grapes (15) Grapefruit Lemon (unlimited) Limes (unlimited) Orange (1) Nectarine (1) Tangerine (1) Apricots (fresh) Papaya Pineapple Fresh figs (2-3) Persimmon (½) Rhubarb	Rice: brown rice, wild, brown basmati, rice noodles Millet Amaranth Teff Quinoa Barley Whole wheat pasta Rye Bulger Oat (steel cut oatmeal) Buckwheat Spelt Kamut Sprouted grain/rye/whole wheat bread (1 slice) Whole grain bagel (½) Whole grain crackers (e.g. Mary's) approximately 10 or 100 calories Popcorn

3 SERVINGS/DAY	2 SERVINGS/DAY	1 SERVING/DAY
HEALTHY FAT: 1 SERVING = 1 TBSP. OR OTHERWISE MARKED	NUTS AND SEEDS (RAW): 1 SERVING = 1 TBSP. OR OTHERWISE MARKED	LEGUMES: 1 SERVING=½ CUP
Extra virgin olive oil Flax seeds (and oil) Chia seeds Avocado (¼) (and oil) Walnut oil Olives (any) Coconut oil Grape seed oil	Almonds (whole) 10 Walnuts (whole) 7 Natural nut butter (any) Sesame seeds Pumpkin seeds Sunflower seeds Cashews 7 Peanuts Hazelnuts 10 Pecans halves 7 Pistachios	Split peas Lentils Chickpeas/garbanzo beans Kidney beans Pinto beans Lima beans Black beans Black eyed peas Navy beans Cannellini beans Mung beans Hummus (¼ cup) Edamame (1 cup unshelled)

3 SERVINGS/DAY	1 SERVING/DAY
VEGETABLES: UNLIMITED	**ROOT VEGETABLE: 1 SERVING = ½ CUP**
Bell pepper (red, orange, green)	Carrots
Asparagus	Parsnips
Cabbage	Rutabaga
Brussels sprouts	Yukon gold potatoes
Okra	Yams
Mushrooms	Sweet potatoes
Tomato	Squash (acorn, butternut)
Sprouts: alfalfa, sunflower, etc.	Beets
Radish (including diakon)	Turnip
Eggplant	
Jalapeno peppers	
Kohlrabi	
Sea vegetables: nori, kelp, wakame, kombu,	
Dulse	
Zucchini	
Spaghetti squash, Acorn squash	
Shallots	
Water chestnuts	
Carrots	
Cauliflower	
Greens: kale, romaine, red lettuce, radicchio,	
endive, spinach, mustard, watercress,	
dandelion, arugula, chicory	
Beans (green and yellow)	
Cucumber	
Fennel	
Onions, Radishes, Leeks	
Celery	
Peas: Sugar snap and snow	
SPICES AND HERBS: (UNLIMITED)	**DAIRY AND ALTERNATIVES: (OPTIONAL): 1 SERVING = ½ CUP OR OTHERWISE MARKED**
Dill, chive, thyme, sage, oregano, licorice, fennel, rosemary, coriander, bay, mint, parsley, basil and more	Almond milk
	Coconut milk
	Hemp milk
	Rice milk
Sea salt, pepper, garlic, paprika, ginger, mustard, cardamom, cayenne, nutmeg, saffron, clove, red pepper flakes, turmeric, cinnamon, cumin and more	Soy milk
	*all unsweetened
	Cow's milk
	Baby bell cheese (1)
	Laughing cow (1)
	Goat cheese (1 oz)
	Feta cheese (1 oz)
	Mozzarella cheese (1)
	Parmesan cheese (1 oz)

ACCEPTABLE CONDIMENTS

USE AS DESIRED, UNLESS SPECIFIED

Hot sauce
Mustard
Ketchup (1 tbsp)
Mayonnaise
BBQ sauce (1 tbsp)
Teriyaki sauce (1 tbsp)
Horseradish
Soda water
Capers
Sundried tomato
Pesto
Salad dressings made with olive oil
Herbal teas

Healthy Condiment Replacements:

Traditionally, condiments have been associated with sugars, preservatives and all around processed ingredients. Why not sub out these empty calories for nutrient dense alternatives?

Consider these:

- Replace bottled dressings with lemon and olive oil. Avoid poor quality oils like vegetable oils, peanut and soybean. Use lemon instead! It's amazing for your liver and helps with detoxification.

- Replace mayonnaise with avocado or hummus; both provide a fresh, vitamin-rich alternative to the stale flavour of mayonnaise.

- Replace ketchup with salsa. Ketchup is high in sugar and contains unnecessary preservatives we can all do without. Sub this out for the tangy flavour of fresh salsa.

Hey! How are you doing? Are any of the following happening?

Are you starting to waver?

Are you reading this book only instead of calling yourself to action?

Are your feelings of fear creeping in?

Are you anxious?

Then choose another option.

YOU always have choice.

Remember this?

Do You Need A Push? We Are Here To Help!

Option #1 Food-Based Accountability

If you are someone who needs that extra little bit of support and accountability in the food department, this is for you!

What you get:

Individualized support from me, Michelle, your nutritionist!

Weekly accountability to help you achieve Your Weight Loss G-Spot

A personalized review of food logs, plus comments for improvements

Peace of mind, knowing that you're making awesome decisions!

Want to know more? Contact Michelle at michelle@strongnutritionandweightloss.com

Option #2 Own It In My Soul Accountability

If you've been nodding your head in recognition and agreement throughout this book so far, but haven't started your journey yet, it's time for some coaching that will kick start your head and your heart into action!

What you get:

Six individual coaching sessions from me, Nancy, your Connection Coach

Daily accountability check-ins (as needed)

This book's content, customized to your individual needs through coaching

The support of someone who gets it, with the ability to help you overcome self-created hurdles

Want to know more? Contact Nancy at Nancy@nancymilton.ca

Below you will find a sample meal plan based on all the parameters listed above that I've created for you.

You decide how you use the sample meal plan. Try to follow it or use it to construct your own. Make sure you like the foods you are eating, because this is hopefully how you will continue to eat after you finish reading this book.

I strongly encourage that you do this and alternate between three to four weekly menus. Doing this will ensure that not only you have lots of variety, but also that your weekly grocery list is then already planned. All you need to do is prep and follow along!

* Remember, if you weigh over 150 lb., please add an extra protein (from the list above) to one of your snacks.

** If you follow this for two weeks and are still finding yourself hungry, please add in a fourth protein, even if you are under 150 lb.

*** This meal plan is intended to show you that variety is possible, despite a few restrictions on grain products like breads, crackers, pasta, etc. You don't have to follow this to the letter; just ensure you're getting all the foods from each category each day.

	DAY 1	DAY 2	DAY 3	DAY 4	DAY 5	DAY 6	DAY 7
B R E A K F A S T	½ cup fruit (cut up) topped with 3 tbsp. hemp and ¼ cup granola (see recipe)	Paleo pancake with the nut butter (see recipe) topped with cinnamon and 2 tbsp. sliced almonds	Tropical twist smoothie (see recipe)	2 eggs any style served over spinach with 1 slice of toast topped with ¼ avocado	Raspberry almond smoothie (see recipe)	Cottage cheese (½ cup) topped with fresh peach (or any fruit) and 1 tbsp. unsweetened coconut and ½ tsp. vanilla extract + ¼ cup bran buds and 2 tbsp. sesame or pumpkin seeds	¾ cup plain Greek yogurt 0% topped with ½ cup of raspberries and sprinkled with 1 tbsp. unsweetened coconut and 2 tbsp. bran buds (optional)
S N A C K	6 Mary's crackers topped with 1 tbsp. natural peanut butter with veggies and ¼ cup hummus	½ portion quest bar and 12 baby carrots	¼ cup Savory Sage white bean dip (see recipe) and any green, yellow or red veggies	¼ cup plain Greek yogurt with ½ cup berries and cinnamon topped with 2 tbsp. pumpkin seeds	1 apple and 1 tbsp. peanut butter	¼ avocado sprinkled with sea salt + 2 tbsp. sunflower seeds	12 Mary's crackers and 12 baby carrots and white bean dip

	DAY 1	DAY 2	DAY 3	DAY 4	DAY 5	DAY 6	DAY 7
L U N C H	Power smoothie + side salad with any veggies (1 tsp. olive oil)	Homemade turkey chili with raw veggies and a slice of bread on the side	veggie wrap (½ cup beans (any), ¼ avocado, any veggies) + ½ cup beet salad (see recipe)	1 can tuna topped over greens salad with a lemon, 2 tsp. olive oil dressing	Vegetable Protein Soup (see recipe) add ½ cup beans (any) and veggies on the side if you would like	1 Ryvita cracker topped with thin spread of light cream cheese and 3-4 oz lox + roasted beet salad	Greek salad (with 1 oz. feta cheese and 1 tsp, olive oil) topped with grilled chicken
S N A C K	3-4 walnuts and 1 baby bell or string cheese	Edamame (unshelled 1 ½ cups) and 8 olives	2 hardboiled eggs with sea salt +2 servings of nuts or seeds	½ cup plain Greek yogurt with ½ cup berries and vanilla extract and 12 almonds	½ cup cottage cheese topped with sea salt and pepper and fresh tomato on the side (and fresh basil if you have it) +10 Mary's crackers or 1 Ryvita cracker	½ cup fruit salad (see recipe) + ¼ cup hummus and veggies (no root veggies)	¼ cup pistachios and 1 fruit

	DAY 1	DAY 2	DAY 3	DAY 4	DAY 5	DAY 6	DAY 7
D I N N E R	Grilled fish (any) + ½ medium sweet potato + grilled zucchini topped with ¼ diced avocado	Chicken stuffed with 1oz goat cheese, sundried tomato served over grilled bok choy (halved) and peppers (brush with 2 tsp. olive oil and balsamic vinegar after cooking)	5-6 large shrimp grilled with garlic and chili flakes served over warm onion spinach salad (see instructions below)	½ cup chickpea sautéed with minimal olive oil with onion, peppers and broccoli (add spices like cumin, paprika, chili, curry), sauté until vegetables are cooked through, serve over cooked spaghetti squash - see instructions	Frittata (see recipe) topped with ¼ avocado and a side of baby carrots	White fish sautéed with lemon served over caramelized onions and peas drizzled with 1 tsp. olive oil once cooked	"Spaghetti" (use kelp or shirataki noodles (any amount) instead of pasta) with any tomato based sauce (add ground chicken or turkey), ½ cup beans per serving and lots of veggies
W A T E R & O T H E R L I Q U I D S							

	DAY 1	DAY 2	DAY 3	DAY 4	DAY 5	DAY 6	DAY 7
SHOPPING LIST FOR THE WEEK	Hemp Granola ingredients (see resources & references section at end of book) Fresh or frozen berries Mary's crackers Natural nut butter Hummus Vegetables Olive oil Protein powder Leaf lettuce Walnuts String or Babybel cheese Fish Sweet potato Avocado Zucchini	Eggs Baking soda Banana Cinnamon Sliced almonds Quest bar Carrots Ingredients for chili resources section Frozen edamame Olives Chicken Goat cheese Sundried tomato (in oil) Bok choy	Ingredients for smoothie in resources section Coconut oil Coconut milk, almond or hemp milk (unsweetened) Ingredients for white bean dip in resources section Pita or tortilla wrap Beet salad ingredients in resources section Eggs Shrimp Nuts (your choice)	Loaf of Ezekiel or Stonemill bread Spinach Plain Greek 0% yogurt Can of tuna Pumpkin seeds Lemon Vanilla extract Chickpeas Broccoli Spaghetti squash Spices like turmeric, curry, cumin and paprika	Smoothie ingredients in resources section Apples Soup ingredients in resources section Cottage cheese Tomato Frittata ingredients in resources section	Coconut (unsweetened) Smoked salmon Cream cheese White fish Frozen peas	Feta Kelp or shirataki noodles Pistachios (raw) Canned beans

Recipes: See References and Resources for recipes from this meal plan

Substitutions

Vegetarians: again, I did not forget about you! I tried to incorporate vegan and vegetarian friendly meals in here (catering to everyone in a week-long plan is quite the challenge).

If there is a food you do not eat (chicken, for example), then sub that food out for something else in the same category that you do eat, like hemp seeds or tofu. For those with food allergies and sensitivities, please consider the same rule of thumb.

I feel compelled, after presenting this chapter, to reiterate what I have already said. Change is hard! I know I'm asking you to do something different, to live your life differently.

Although, at the beginning, this might prove challenging, I can say with certainty: within only a short time, this will NO LONGER seem new or difficult.

It will simply just be the way you live your life—and you'll find a happier, healthier and ultimately lighter, amazing YOU!

Enjoy! Remember that you need to like these foods you are eating or this won't stick. Once you're comfortable with the phases, then we can start to introduce new recipes and variety to your diet.

FREE BONUS RESOURCES

Want to learn more? Maybe you want to print out the charts from this chapter? Go ahead! We have created a free membership area where you have access to other valuable bonus resources. http://bonus.weightlossgspot.com/

Chapter 7: Keys to G

- The 3:2:1 G Pillar system was developed only if you've already moved through other skills and activities in the book. Before you tackle this stage, make sure you're ready.

- Pillar 1 is your removal stage. This will last ONE week and it consists of eliminating those "foods" that hinder your ability to think straight and lose fat! These are obvious sugars, hidden sources of sugar and white flours/grains.

- Pillar 2 is your "rules" phase. Pillar 2 and 3 will happen simultaneously and last until you reach your goal. Make sure you read, understand and follow these rules while constructing your meal plans and consuming from your G-Spot friendly foods list.

- Pillar 3 includes your specific instructions about what and how much to eat. Please ensure you are having ALL the foods listed (no more and no less).

- Enjoy! Remember that you need to like these foods you are eating or this won't stick. Once you're comfortable with the phases, then we can start to introduce new recipes and variety to your diet.

8

SHHHH! I'M HUNTING MY G-SPOT

Nancy here again!

I'm 42 years old, and for the first 36 years of my life, I was unaware of the concept of self-talk.

Or maybe I knew I was self-talking, but I wasn't familiar with the term. Or maybe I wasn't aware that I was self-talking and just thought this is just what went on in my head and how I treated myself.

Any which way, it wasn't until my mid-30s, sitting in a coaching training course, that the idea of self-talk was introduced to me in the form of an idea called "saboteur."

At the time, I was hearing the term saboteur often (it may have been my age, it may have been my career niche, it may have been because I was talking about it and becoming more aware of it), and it was a good thing.

To be happier and healthier, we all need to be aware of our own self-talk. I'm going to share my spin on your self-talk with you and how it relates to this amazing journey you are on.

There are two areas from which our thoughts seem to develop, and I am not referring to left and right brain or top and bottom brain.

I'm referring to the positive and negative areas that your thoughts come from.

I picture them as positive and negative thought boxes in my head. This may surprise you, but we need both positive and negative thoughts to live and to function. Consider what you would do from a reaction standpoint without negative feelings like fear, fright or anger. These "watch out" feelings help move you to respond to specific situations, steering you away from harm.

For example, a sense of danger may move you to action if you smelled smoke in your home at 2:30 a.m. Without this negative response, you might not get out of the bed and take care of yourself and others in your home!

Having awareness of the amount of positive and negative emotion you host in your head daily is helpful.

But you also need to think about how long you host a negative emotion before you allow it to breed and then fester into harmful saboteur or self-talk. I suggest you allow a maximum of 10 seconds to process a healthy negative indicator.

That's enough time to consider and create momentum to take care of you in this situation. What does this mean? The longer a negative thought continues in our mind, the longer we are allowing it to control or impact our behaviour, influence our confidence, and distract us from who we really are.

To recap:

Positive, real thoughts = okay

Negative, judging thoughts that last longer than 10 seconds = not okay

(for example: "I suck, I suck, I suck, I suck, I SUUUUUUUCCCCCCKKKKK")

These positive and negative areas develop in our minds throughout our life, beginning in early childhood. This is important to state, because sometimes they may have been with us for as long as we can consciously remember.

On numerous occasions when I have acknowledged a client's saboteur or negative self-talk, they aren't even aware of what I'm referring to because that's all they know and remember. Some negative self-talk voices have been with us for most of our lives. They're like emotional files stored in our subconscious brain that we access without even realizing we have them. Ugh.

Some of us hear only one inner voice in our head and others have more than one. Truth be told, it doesn't matter if you have one, or if you have seven. What matters is that you're aware of them. Then you can take action to make the unconstructive voices quieter and decide to hear from them less and less.

These inner voices hold as much power as you grant them. In other words, they can be pretty darn powerful! I'll let you guess who controls them. YEP, that would be you.

It's time to figure this out and the time is now.

A disclaimer: from everything I've read and researched regarding saboteurs, my understanding is that there is no magic way to get rid of them.

This chapter will help you identify your saboteurs, discover how to identify their cues, provide some action examples to shrink them and lastly, challenge you to build a plan to keep them small.

Identification

First, we need to know what we're dealing with.

You may have read the first page of this chapter and thought to yourself, "I'm not following. What the heck are Nancy and Michelle talking about?"

We need to figure out how much self-talk you currently have breeding within you so that we can devise a plan to shut those negative voices up.

Here are some personal examples of self-talk, straight from my clients:

- "You're fat."

- "You're never going to lose weight, so quit trying."

- "You suck. You failed AGAIN today."

- "You will always be big."

- "Just start tomorrow."

- "You've screwed up today already, why not just keep eating?"

- "You can't do this. You've never pulled this off before."

- "You're lazy."

- "You're not worth it."

- "You're so lame."

- "You can't do anything right."

- "You're not good enough"

CRAZY talk, yes?

There is NO WAY we would ever speak to someone else like this.

Yet we speak to ourselves in our heads—constantly. And then we wonder why we're aren't successful!

For the next seven days, we'll be conducting what I like to call Awareness Week.

Your job is to carry a pad of sticky notes and a pen with you wherever you go.

Anytime you have a thought that's specifically negative toward the way you feel about you, record what your self-talk voice said.

Then take a moment to capture the feeling that this voice provoked. If you need inspiration, look to the examples above. One thought per sticky, please.

By the end of the week you may have 50 sticky notes—or 350. This exercise is not about the number of sticky notes you have. It's about tracing and tracking the negativity going on inside your head.

There's also a chance that your inner voice calls you names. Because, of course, slamming you with one-liner ridicule is not enough.

Have you ever heard the voice in your head launch bully tosses like:

- Lazybones

- Suck

- Worthless

- Ugly girl

- Gross

- Fatty

- Pudgy

- Chubbo

- Rolypoly

If your inner voice is a name-caller, versus a one-line axe-thrower, write those examples down, too.

Doesn't matter what kind of bully lives in your head—they're all mean, hurtful, and debilitating. If anyone spoke to my children this way, I am very clear how I would handle that situation!

Yet we harass ourselves like this daily, and then expect that we can easily change lifelong habits based on this ridicule.

Cuckoo, don't you think?

Let's just recap: you have one week to record the various names your inner voice calls you as well as any one-liners your inner voice tosses your way. Use as many sticky notes as you want.

BUT you must record these statements in the moment. See you in 7 days.

Okay, welcome back! Good to have you here. Quite the week of awareness. YOWser. But it was a step we needed for the process. Now, it's time for...

Part Two Of Identification

It's been a week. You have a stack of sticky notes that are hurtful, mean and ugly.

It's time to figure out your theme(s).

STEP 1 Sort It Out!

1. Lay your sticky notes in front of you individually

2. Review them and consider any patterns or themes you notice, like similar messages in the same voice (for example, my Grade Two teacher's voice saying, "You're fat!")

3. Clump those nasty saboteur notes with the themes you've identified.

4. Transfer the themes to a separate piece of paper and answer these questions per theme. A suggestion: write out the answer so you see and feel it more deeply.

- How long have you been hearing that annoying inner voice? Think about it, and summarize, how that voice controls you daily?

- Now, think about who powers this voice.

- Outline specifically: how will keeping this voice around benefit you?

- Define three WOWie ways your life would be different if this voice was muted.

5. Breathe. Reread your answers. Consider and mourn what you have been doing to yourself! Please treat yourself with kindness and wholeheartedness in this step (and always). You've got to fully let this go to be able to move forward in a healthy way. Treat yourself lovingly and with care. xo

6. Like the burning exercise we completed a few chapters ago, we encourage you to either shred or burn (think bonfire!) these awful sticky notes. Release those destructive thoughts, please!

STEP 2 Identify The Cues

Let's move on.

Now you have a list of all the inner voice, mean girl names you've been dealing with. You know that those voices are harming the way you're living and influencing your happiness.

If you're unclear at this point, go back to Step 1 and answer the questions—for real this time!

It's time to have courage and make some changes.

Here we go! Let's start at the beginning:

1. Review your themes. Consider when each theme occurs.

For example, coming out of the shower and drying yourself in the mirror may be your "look at all the things that are wrong with my body," daily routine.

OR it could be that, while you're showering, you're saying to yourself, "I don't have it in me to eat well today. I suck."

I'd call the first theme "Naked Mirror Bully Talk" and the second "My glass is half empty".

2. Record your theme(s) based on the time of day, your mood and the kind of day you've had: high stress, completing repetitive, redundant tasks, etc.

3. What provokes your inner voice to chime in? This could range from choosing an outfit in the morning and finding your clothes aren't fitting properly, to any time you go to make a food or meal choice.

4. Prioritize, by impact, which theme seems to push you harder and faster into a downward spiral.

STEP 3 Action

We've already talked about the difference between awareness and action.

Awareness was Step One and Two.

Welcome to Step Three!

We can have awareness until the cows come home. But awareness will give us squat if we don't take action!

It's common knowledge that more people than not break their New Year's resolution by the last day in January because they've fumbled their action plan.

The plan is the key—and this is a fumble-free book.

It's time for more change. Let's do this!

Choosing your top priority from Step 2, consider the reverse of the downward spiral your negative inner voice has created. Make a specific list of what those could be.

Here's an example:

"Any time I'm eating well, my inner voice—all day long—sings the 'Give me something sweet' refrain. Thoughts like, 'I can't go on without a cookie,' 'I must have_____,' 'Just have one! You can start tomorrow,' and/or 'You look okay, so come on, eat what you deserve,' etc."

If/when (and who are we kidding? There's always a when!) that negative voice chimes in, we've started a list for you on actionable ideas to reverse an inevitable downward spiral into the negativity abyss.

Use the ones that fit for you, edit them for your needs, or make more. It doesn't matter.

Make a list of ten (positive) affirmations on the effort you are making. For example:

- "I can do this."

- "It feels WOWie when I do the right thing for me!"

- "I've got this."

- "Time to own the change I want for myself."

This is important: Create a specific "why this is important to me" list.

- Preset your menu for the day an ensure you choose items you look forward to eating

- Write a jingle for yourself to sing: "I rock because I can stick to my goals. La la la!"

- Remove ALL possible food traps

- Record your two lists and carry them with you

- Start every morning with intentions for the day

- Place your hand on your heart and ask yourself, "What does my heart feel (in this moment)?"

- Change your usual routine. For example, "I'll only go to Starbucks when I'm meeting a client. If I go on my own, I know will lose control and buy a dessert."

- When that voice comes up, turn the volume down. Literally visualize a dimmer switch and turn the light from high to low

- Record your old habit on a piece of paper. Stick it in an outdoor fire and let it burn. Release it! It's not yours anymore

- Set a timer for 15 minutes and then check in with "Do I really need this?"

- Ask yourself in the moment: "Am I hungry or is this my inner voice talking?"

- Breathe

- Ignore your inner voice. Because every time you give it a consideration, it's like adding fuel to the fire

Check out the list above and circle three action plans you're going to apply.

Then, at the beginning of each day, review the top three "reverse of the spiral" and create a "what to do in the moment" to stop yourself from listening to that dumb inner voice. Make a pact with yourself!

At the end of each day, record what you did well to slow the self-talk and what one thing you need to do differently tomorrow to get better at it.

*Repeat this process for every theme

STEP 4 Shrink It

We're all human. We've all experienced self-talk.

But those who defeat it have learned to shrink it. The power of shrinkage is the power of control. Ever skinny-dipped with a man? Ha!

Remind me who has control here. Mmmm hmmmm. That would be you!

You get to choose how you run your life, make decisions, and take on your day, right? So you now get to decide IF you want this voice to continue in your head.

Here are a couple of visuals that may assist you when you hear that inner voice:

Picture the positive and negative boxes I told you about at the beginning of this chapter.

For me the positive box is green, the negative box is red. Any time I hear from the inner voice, it's like the negative box heats up. Using one of my actions, I visualize me throwing positive (green) onto the red box, like putting the fire or flame out.

Then laugh your cartoon character crazy laugh and say "Bhahahahah! Be gone, negative voice!" It's amazing how humour and context can diffuse any situation.

1. Ask yourself: "Who's making the decisions today? Bully witch or ME?"

2. Tell your inner voice, "You're not the boss of me. Go away!"

3. Or _____. Insert ANY idea here that makes you feel good and shifts your perspective.

Chapter 8 Keys to G

- We all self-talk. It's how you handle yours that is key.

- When it's positive, self-talk is a wonderful tool that can help you succeed in any and all aspects of life. But when it's negative, it can be soul crushing.

- This chapter is the key to your realization of what can happen when you listen acutely to the NEGATIVE self-talk and the daily damage it's doing.

- You get to choose the voice you listen to and how to handle it or turn it to low or off. Learn now and be consistent with it, and you win!

DOWNLOAD YOUR FREE WORKBOOK

Remember to download the free Workbook. We created PDF's so you can print them out and use as you are working your way through the book. This will aid greatly in your success!

Get access to your free bonus resources at
http://bonus.weightlossgspot.com/

9

THE MISSIONARY POSITION

Hey, it's Nancy for a chapter on keeping things spicy!

Vanilla ice cream.

A blank sheet of paper.

A beige room.

A gray t-shirt.

The missionary position.

Read that list again. One more time, now. Yawning yet? While there's nothing intrinsically wrong with any of these things, you have to admit that it's a pretty ho-hum collection of nondescript items. So, why am I asking you examine this lame list? Your job is to notice what all these things have in common. Once you do, you'll understand what this phase of your weight-loss journey is all about.

Be careful not to cop out by simply telling me that all these things are boring. That's too easy. What else can you say about them? Think about how these things make you feel. Personally, for me, they're neutral. I feel neither here nor there about them. Interesting...

Interesting that some things, like the stuff in my list, represent neutral territory. These simple things just are what they are. We accept that. But we also know that any of these items could potentially be the basis for something pretty awesome...basis being the operative word. All they need to get to the next level is a tweak, addition or enhancement.

You know, some bells and whistles:

Smother the ice cream with sprinkles and caramel sauce and you've got ecstatic kids.

Fold the paper like origami and wow a friend with an original art piece.

Add patterned curtains, bold furniture and bright paintings to the boring walls and you've created a beautiful, energetic space.

Transform the plain t-shirt into a head-turning outfit by popping on a vintage scarf and statement earrings.

Start out in the missionary position for some foreplay and then move on to... (insert your imaginative ideas here)!

Here's the point. When things become too familiar, too expected, too ho-hum, it's time to take it up a notch. That's what we're doing here in Chapter 9. Taking it up a notch! The "missionary-position phase" of weight-loss is fine; but it's often an indication that it's time for something more.

About The Plateau

Here's another analogy for you. Let's think for a minute about that delicious stage in a relationship when we're just beginning to date someone new. The dreamy honeymoon phase. You know what I'm talking about... So exciting. So fresh. If you've been with your guy for a while, think back, way back. (If you're in this phase now, enjoy every minute!)

TRADEMARKS OF THE HONEYMOON PHASE
On very best behaviour.
Spending a lot of time getting dressed, wearing favourite/most flattering outfits.
Rereading emails/texts before sending to make sure message is absolutely perfect.
Extra attention to perfumes, colognes, deodorants, lip balms, moisturizers, etc.
Minty gum always on hand.
Feeling positive and energized because of the attention of a new guy!

Believe it or not, it's possible to make a direct correlation from the above list to your weight-loss journey. What's that, you say? Dating can't possibly have anything in common with dieting? Wrong. Read the list below, and try to tell me you can't relate. (I know you can!)

TRADEMARKS - RELATIONSHIP HONEYMOON PHASE	TRADEMARKS – WEIGHT LOSS HONEYMOON PHASE
On best behaviour.	You record every morsel you eat, including when you ate it and size of meal.
Spending a lot of time getting dressed, wearing favourite/most flattering outfits.	You keep trying on that special outfit you're striving to fit into. You notice it's starting to fit! You're happy about feeling and looking better in it.
Examining/editing emails and texts before sending to make sure messages are absolutely perfect.	You examine each bite of food before consuming it, and write daily in your food journal about what you can do differently to optimize success.
Extra attention to perfumes, colognes, deodorants, lip balms, moisturizers, etc.	You pay extra attention to meal preparation; you experiment with new recipes and try new foods.
Minty gum always on hand.	You always have prepared meals and pre-arranged snacks on hand so that you don't succumb to impulse eating.
Feeling positive and energized because of the attention of a new guy!	You feel positive because you're focusing on you. You notice that your smart choices are impacting how you feel, and you're energized about "taking on" your life!

It's true, dating and dieting share commonalities. Enthusiasm, excitement and novelty are all colliding to motivate you in both situations. Let's talk about dating some more and see if there are other lessons to be drawn.

You're six months into the dating relationship. If you've stayed with this person it's probably because you're liking him more and more. At the same time, you're growing to know him better. As you continue to learn more about your special someone, you begin to see other sides of his personality. If months eventually stretch into years, the lustre of the honeymoon phase is likely to tarnish a bit. Or maybe even a lot! That said, there are some couples out there who do a great job of keeping some of that honeymoon feeling alive. What are some things that these couples do to keep things fresh?

Here are a few habits of couples in successful long-term relationships. (Yes, this is a weight-loss book... but isn't it handy that we provide relationship tips as well? No extra charge!)

- Date night (once a week/month)

- Regular vacations

- Staycations (with parameters like no chores, no technology, etc.)

- Daily dinner table share of "rose and thorn" of the day (aka, "highs and lows")

- Embrace the never-go-to-bed-angry-with-each-other rule

- Love messages (cards, post-it note surprises on the steering wheel of the car, a hand-written poem or even a naughty text)

- Breakfast in bed

- Creating reminder list of "I love you because…"

- Sharing favourite memories from relationship

You might have some favourites to add to the list too. The point is, you need to mix it up! Same old, same old, can get, well… old! Everyone knows that monotony can be the kiss of death when trying to keep the spark in a relationship alive. Now think about your past dieting habits. Are they monotonous? See where I'm going with this…?

Michelle here: Just like uninspired relationships, dieting (in the traditional sense of the word) can lack lustre and become boring and repetitive. I'd get sick of eating nothing but steamed broccoli and boiled chicken too! But remember, what we are doing here is not a diet. It's a WOWie, change-your-mind-and-body lifestyle transformation. Aren't transformations are supposed to be new and exciting? I think so!

With my clients, I always encourage them to change things up as much as possible. I don't want them falling into their old familiar patterns of bland, tasteless diet foods. New recipes are one way to shake things up a bit. I have lots of other suggestions too. Keep reading to check out many ways to keep your transformation process feeling fresh and positive.

If you do hit that point in your weight-loss journey where everything feels kind of beige, or vanilla, or missionary position, don't be surprised. Know that for many a plateau is inevitable; one of the best, most powerful things you can do is just keep plugging along until the next breakthrough happens. Sometimes the body needs a bit of a break, just as our minds do from time to time. Giving your body that time will generally kick it back into weight-loss mode within two or three weeks, at most.

However… if you plateau for longer than three weeks, it's time to go back to Week 1 of the program. Just like a boyfriend who starts to take you for granted, sometimes a little kick in the butt is all your body needs to be its best!

You've done a great job reflecting on relationships and weight-loss programs so far. They have a lot in common, particularly in the way that they tend to ebb and flow. Let's recap some key points:

With weight loss, like in dating, there are points where we may hit plateaus.

Learning to accept this kind of rhythm (the ups and downs) and even learn to expect the plateaus, sets us up for success.

It's valuable to prepare for that inevitable moment when we hit a plateau. Be prepared with specific ideas and activities to "mix it up."

Under The Microscope

Here's another way in which your weight-loss program might remind you of your relationship challenges. Often with weight loss there's a lot of scrutiny going on. You do want to be conscientious and careful with your weight-loss program; but just as too much scrutiny can kill the mojo when dating, so too it is with dieting. Remember Jerry Seinfeld? His girlfriend's always had some little thing wrong with them: close talker, weird laugh… If he hadn't scrutinized things so much, maybe some of those fleeting romances could have blossomed.

Whether you call it "under the microscope," "the magnifying-glass effect" or "looking through the fish bowl," extreme scrutiny is something to beware of on your journey. We often assess our own weight-loss situation through a critical lens, and more often than not that lens is not objective. Typically, we've been judging our weight through this same warped lens for years—this is a well-trained, if not accurate, lens! Most of us have created a set of expectations by which we judge ourselves, and for a bunch of reasons we've become pretty good at upping the expectations over time.

With that in mind, let's explore two areas related to the "missionary position" or plateau phase of your weight-loss program:

1) You're potentially judging yourself harder on this effort than on anything else in your life. Imagine if someone were critiquing your every move in the bedroom! How do you think that would affect your results in that arena? Yikes. Likewise, too much criticism will stifle your weight-loss success.

> *Michelle here: Oooh the stories I've heard! Ladies, you are so hard on yourselves! Pretend you are listening to your best friend when you hear that voice. Would you insult and drag her down as you have done to yourself? I think not. If you are plateauing, be patient with yourself.*

2) Now is the time to ask yourself: What, specifically, can I start doing now (both today and moving forward) to hit my weight-loss stride? Let's figure out what you are going to do right here, right now to break your old habits. How can you get out from under the same old "missionary position" and get on top of your choices, your health (and your man!).

Here's the good news: you're reading Chapter 9. That means you've already learned a lot about how your perspective may have contributed to the nature of your particular lens. You should have some awareness about the way your lens is colouring the way you think about your plateau or missionary position phase.

Reflect on that fact while you try to get a healthy, accurate perspective on your current level of success.

If you feel like you're still judging yourself and unhealthy scrutiny continues to hold you back, I encourage you to repeat Chapter 8. Another strategy would be to sign up for some coaching. (Ideally with me!)

Pulling It All Together

Let's reflect on what you've read so far in this chapter. In your romantic life, you probably know how to handle the missionary position with ease; maybe you even find enjoyment here. Yes, it can create a bird's nest hairstyle while doing it; but nonetheless, personally, I've learned to adapt and ride it out with pleasure! The question now is this: will you apply this same laid-back attitude to the "missionary-position phase" of weight loss? How are you going to handle your plateau?

To answer that question, let's start out by imagining ourselves in a bedroom situation. Think about how you'd ideally like the missionary position (a plateau) to feel. Below are twenty-four feelings that might describe the experience. Read them and circle your five favourites. Feel free to add your own words if you think of better ones!

READ AND CIRCLE YOUR FIVE FAVOURITE FEELINGS			
Comforting	Protected	Engaged	Dedicated
Relaxing	Soothing	Confident	Connected
Devoted	Easy	Focused	Assured
At ease	Self-aware	Self-regard	Powerful
Tranquil	Believable	Committed	Calm
Safe	Tenacious	Faithful	Secure

To demonstrate how this works, I'm going to choose five random words from the list:

- Easy

- Tranquil

- Powerful

- Engaged

- Confident

Michelle here: I want to play too! Here are my words: Powerful, Committed, Ease, Self-aware, Calm

Ummhmmm… when I read my five words together, my mind goes to a happy place. Together they paint a picture of a very satisfying romp. Think about your words. How does your imagined experience sound? Good, right? I thought so! The missionary position isn't so bad, so blah, when you put your mind in the right place, is it?

Now you need to figure out a way to feel good about the weight-loss version of the missionary position too.

Before reading this chapter you might have had some less-than positive feelings attached to this phase. Is any of this self-talk familiar to you?

- What is wrong with me? Why am I stuck in this plateau?

- Poor me! I've worked my tail off only to land here forever in this "middle ground."

- I don't even know what I want. Why am I doing this again?

To move away from these kinds of self-defeating thoughts about the missionary-position phase, try applying your list of feeling words. Make a connection between the words you circled and the plateau state that you're in; this should enhance your awareness about what's actually going on here in this stage. One of the many mottos I use with my clients is: "Awareness and Action!" It's time for you to activate this motto for yourself.

For me, easy, tranquil, powerful, engaged, and confident mean: "I've got this." Thinking "I've got this" makes me stabilize where I'm at and manage my self-talk. These feelings remind me that I can choose how to respond to any situation. They also give me a clearer perspective on the missionary-position phase when it comes to weight loss. When I think about this stage now, I have thoughts such as:

- Just go with it.

- It's part of the journey.

- It's the opposite of a negative thing.

- Your body is adjusting and stabilizing to some of the positive changes you are making for yourself.

- Rome wasn't built in a day.

Plateaus have a tendency to make us feel impatient and frustrated, but try not to let this happen. The next time you feel impatient, just stop for a moment and ask yourself this question: Would I rather be at this place (my plateau) or where I was before I started this weight-loss program? I thought so. So stay here then. Embrace your body, making the adjustments it needs to for this transformation to be a long-term one for you. A WOWie one!

How Long Is Too Long?

"Okay," you may be thinking to yourself. "I can be patient. I can wait this out." Careful! This is not a true "I've got this" perspective. Why? Because it's lacking two key circled qualities, namely powerful and confident. Patience is important but it's not the only quality to focus on in this phase. You need to be able to answer this question for yourself: How long is too long in the missionary position?

If you are stuck in a mode with only patience, but still can't get out of this tired old missionary or plateau position, move back half a page and take the time to OWN IT IN YOUR SOUL. Yes, you deserve that let-loose, unbridled WOWser bedroom sex! Oh, wait, this is a weight loss book… I mean you also deserve to get the thrill of seeing the pounds melt away and your skinny jeans and favourite dress fit better.

Change The Equation

Years ago I was watching Oprah's daily show and a now well-known expert by the name of Dr. Phil was on the episode as a special guest. The theme of the show had something to do with finding Mr. Right. The panel featured five single women. Each had a solid education and career, was physically fit and attractive, and owned a home. Their question for Dr. Phil was: What am I doing wrong?

Dr. Phil explained: "It's not that you're doing anything wrong, yet something in the equation is not allowing you to meet men that you want to spend time with. So you need to change your equation."

The reason I'm sharing the Dr. Phil example is to reinforce that well-known definition of insanity, commonly attributed to Albert Einstein:

> *Insanity* = repeating the same action, expecting a different result.

When in the weight-loss missionary position, you're a lot like the Dr. Phil women. They seem to have "all the right stuff." Yet, when the rubber meets the road, they aren't meeting the quality guys they hope for. Dr. Phil's response to them is just like the one I'm now offering you. Ditch your old equation. Face it: it isn't working. It's time to shake things up!

So, stop repeating the same actions over and over if you want a new result. Don't know how to begin your shake-up? Here are a few ideas to get you started...

IF YOU NOW REGULARLY...	TOMORROW TRY...
eat the same thing for breakfast...	an egg white omelette with roasted asparagus and lemon!
walk for 30 minutes after dinner...	jump rope with the kids, a yoga class, or a bike ride with a friend.
enjoy 10 plain almonds for your 3 pm snack...	an apple with almond butter, or how about Mary's crackers with hummus?
always have sex in the missionary position...	anything else!

Michelle here: Don't stop at just switching up what you do. Also think about what time you do it! Even varying the times at which you eat can be helpful. You'd be surprised at how much even small changes can "salsa-fy" things for your system!

You've made it to Chapter 9, so clearly you've done a great job of following your plan to a T. Yet you now find yourself in a plateau. Not a problem. All that means is that your body–mind–spirit (or whatever!) needs to turn that T on its head. Or maybe you don't need a complete about-face—perhaps you just need to twist that T into a different shape! Take a close look at your food journal. Examine your daily routine. Really think about your game plan and get serious about "salsa-fying" it!

Other ideas for shaking things up:

- New recipes: Ask your friends for their favourites. Subscribe to an online foodie blog or to a healthy food magazine for new ideas.

- "This Instead of That": This philosophy can be applied to almost any food choice. For example, try my Island Alive Smoothie instead of your usual berry one (see the Resources and References section at the end of the book for this recipe)

- Be a joiner: Enroll in a new fitness class. Join a walking club. (Bring a friend!) I just joined an improvisation class; it's fun to meet people and it's active.

- Music: A great motivator! Add some new great tunes to your run; change up the rhythms. At the end of each song, add in a quick sprint or ten squats.

- Bust up the rut: Change up any little thing in your daily routine: work out at a different time, eat out instead of bringing in lunch everyday (or vice versa), etc.

- Seek inspiration: Join online food forums or community groups to educate yourself more about new trends in health, fitness, and nutritious foods. Connect with people whom have already had and hold weight loss success. Befriend them. Watch on-line videos. Books work too!

- Clean out: Find a good nutritionist and have her set you up with a safe and structured cleanse or detox.

- Top it up: Try increasing your usual quantities for a week or two. For example, drink more water and/or green tea than your usual intake. Or eat more vegetables per meal than usual. (Warning: do not try this with chocolate!)

- Calorie cycle: Eat slightly more calories on Day 1 and then slightly less on Day 2. Repeat for two weeks.

- Start tracking your food and drink again if you have stopped doing this.

- Congratulate yourself: Mani-pedi! Shopping spree! Weekend getaway!

Whether a big treat or small, make sure you consistently reward yourself for goals met. Acknowledging your progress to yourself or others is celebration in itself. And a reminder: in the past you may have gotten to this plateau, grown frustrated, and eaten your way out. Congratulate yourself on sticking the weight!

Celebrate Your Success

Remember Kool and the Gang? "Ceeeeee-leb-rate good times, come on!" Even though you may be in the missionary position on your weight-loss journey, this is your theme song for this phase. Really.

We know you're serious about setting weight-loss objectives and meeting them. That's part of the reason why your plateau is causing you frustration; your objectives seem elusive right now. Ironically, though, we see your plateau as a cause for celebration. "Come on!"

Hear us out. You've made some significant changes for yourself, right? Some were easy, such as drinking more water and logging your food choices; some were harder, like eating more frequently and adding more protein into your day. Whatever changes you've made, it's important to recognize your accomplishments. It's time now to pause and acknowledge the improvements you've made in your day-to-day life. Let's make a list so you can really see your progress in black and white.

What have you done for yourself to get closer to your lifestyle goals? Be specific.

_____

_____

_____

What impact have these changes brought to your life? How important is it that you keep up these new habits?

_____

_____

_____

We can't see your responses, but we'd be willing to bet that you've created a pretty WOWie list. Knowing that you've dedicated the time to read this book and that you've put an action plan into place, it's likely that you have followed through by making some significant life changes. Yes? However, if your list is anything less than WOWie, get back up there and connect with the questions! If you can't acknowledge and celebrate yourself who the heck else is going to?

Your list (either the first draft or the one you just re-wrote thanks to our coaxing) is a big deal. The reason it's so important is that it shows that you're taking yourself and your health on as a serious priority. Celebrate that. Celebrate the fact that you are being responsible, accountable, and prioritizing the right things in your life. Also, with the work we did on self-talk, this is a great POSITIVE turn around on some of those old habit thoughts.

What could this celebration look like, you wonder? Refer back in Chapter 3 for ideas.

Now, go circle three options for yourself and DO THEM. You deserve it!

GO!

> **Chapter 9: Keys to G**
>
> • The missionary position can be more foundational than we realize. Embrace and respect this inevitable phase — that way it won't feel so **BLAH**. Like the vanilla ice cream under the decadent sundae, use it as your starting point for something even more exciting.
>
> • If you find you're in a rut, it's time to salsa-fy! That goes for this weight-loss process or anything else, for that matter. Changing things up is key to real progress.

Michelle here: When I hear the word "salsa-fy, I picture one of those scantily-clad Hula dancers shaking her money maker. Get a new outfit (a little black dress perhaps?), get moving, do something!

FREE BONUS RESOURCES

Want to learn more? We have created a free membership area where you have access to other valuable bonus resources to will help you dive deeper!

Get access to your free bonus resources at
http://bonus.weightlossgspot.com/

10

I'M NOT IN THE MOOD

Hey, it's Michelle again! Let's talk about stress, baby!

"A man, ninety years old, was asked to what he attributed his longevity.
'I reckon,' he said, with a twinkle in his eye, 'It's because most nights I
went to bed and slept when I should have sat up and worried.' "

— Dorothea Kent

On a scale of 1 to 10, where 1 represents little to no stress and 10
represents high, unbearable, chronic stress, where would you rate
yourself on average through the day?

1	2	3	4	5	6	7	8	9	10

Once you have given yourself a rating, complete the following stress
questionnaire.

Put a check mark beside each description that applies to you:

STRESS QUESTIONNAIRE
PUT A CHECK MARK BESIDE EACH DESCRIPTION THAT APPLIES TO YOU
I get gassy, bloated or experience heartburn through the day, especially after meals.
I have a hard time falling and/or staying asleep.
I wake up tired and unrefreshed.
I have a difficult time losing weight despite changes to diet and lifestyle.
I have belly fat.
I experience cravings for sweet and or salty foods most days.
I have poor muscle tone or have a difficult time building lean muscle mass.
I get dizzy upon standing or kneeling.
I have a general feeling of weakness and fatigue through the day.
I have little or no sex drive.
I have a hard time concentrating; I get distracted easily.
I tend to have low motivation and/or trouble making decisions.
I do not deal with stress well.
I end up with colds and infections easily.
My bowel movements are often either too loose or I'm constipated.
/15 TOTAL

Stress Makes You Fat

In my nutritional practice, one of the first questions I ask new clients is about stress levels. This gives me a sense of their lifestyle, how they cope, how their body is coping with change and how successful they will be with weight loss.

Generally, clients rate their stress levels low to average, or between 1 and 6 on the scale above. Moving along, in a very detailed health assessment, questions similar to the ones above are also addressed; do you have belly fat, do you experience cravings, etc.

I've discovered in my time working with clients, that most people aren't clear what stress is, don't know the symptoms associated with stress and that perhaps they are, in fact, stressed.

It is only when I start connecting the dots that clients start taking a deeper look at their lives and realize that all the little nagging symptoms that contributed to making them feel lousy were largely due to stress.

My theory is that many people claim low stress levels because it's all they know—and so it simply seems normal. How sad! So many people live with chronic stress that they aren't even aware that how they are living and coping is abnormal.

So now that you've rated your stress out of 10 and taken the quiz, here's what I want you to do. Read through the rest of the chapter, see if this information resonates with you, decide if you still want to keep your rating as is, or change it and we will discuss the results of the quiz at the end of the chapter.

Stress, according to the Oxford Dictionary, is "a state of mental or emotional strain or tension resulting from adverse or demanding circumstances."

And guess what? Stress makes you fat!

If you want to stop reading now, that is essentially all I need you to take from this chapter. When you're stressed, your body produces a hormone called cortisol and one of the main functions of cortisol is to signal your body to store fat. This is a survival mechanism built into our genetics from our caveman days—but today, it's wreaking havoc on many of our bodies.

In addition to cortisol production, stress alters the delicate balance of our super important, make-you-feel-sexy-in-the-sack, fat-busting hormones!

G-Spot Lovin' Hormones At-A-Glance:

- Serotonin

- DHEA

- Leptin

- Dopamine

- Melatonin

- GABA

- Thyroid hormones

- Glucagon

- Progesterone

- Adrenalin

- Testosterone

- Growth hormone

Serotonin: fondly dubbed "the happy chemical," is a hormone concentrated in our gastrointestinal systems. Chronic levels of stress interfere with serotonin production, causing mood fluctuations. This can result in carbohydrate cravings because the body tries to regulate itself by increasing blood sugar and therefore, energy. Too many simple carbohydrates can, as we have learned, create issues for people trying to lose weight.

DHEA: a hormone produced by the adrenal glands. It helps regulate fat metabolism and muscle building. Simply put: if your stress levels are always high, it stands to reason that your adrenal glands will always be under pressure to perform. This constant reliance on these organs tires them out, often causing adrenal fatigue. As a result, lower levels of DHEA are produced, which lessens that amazing fat-burning effect we're after.

When **leptin** is functioning optimally, we are better able to regulate our consumption of food. Among other things, leptin allows us to regulate when we are hungry and when we are not. When there is an imbalance of this hormone, some people are triggered to constantly forage for food without really ever feeling satisfied from a meal.

Leptin is primarily released during sleep; however, those under chronic stress are often not getting the restful sleeps they need in order to produce this necessary chemical.

Dopamine: a wonderful neurotransmitter that is released when we partake in pleasurable activities like sex, eating good food and dancing. When we produce enough of this hormone, weight loss can more easily be achieved because dopamine helps to control appetite. Too little can cause overeating, depression and carbohydrate craving.

Interestingly enough, dopamine is produced during times of pleasure and stress. Knowing this, we can better understand why for some people, stress is addictive.

Examples of this could include extreme sports like skydiving and mountain climbing. These sports create a source of stress to the body and therefore, result in a dopamine rush.

Remember though, short bursts of stress are okay. It's long-term, chronic stress that can create health issues.

Melatonin: Do you ever wonder why, in the evening when you should be getting sleepy and ready for bed, you're getting your second wind? And no matter how hard you try, you just can't get to sleep?

Unfortunately, this happens more often than you think. Melatonin is a wonderful gem of a hormone that when it kicks in, makes us feel drowsy in the evening. I have clients that suffer from sleep disturbances on a nightly basis. If you're in the same boat, I feel for you, I really do! Lack or poor quality sleep can be a huge contributor to your weight loss woes.

During the wee hours of the night is when your body is building and preparing all the right hormones and chemicals needed for optimal fat burn. If you miss out on this sleep, you miss out on these vital weight loss powerhouses.

Tip: Sleep like a baby

The benefits of sleep are innumerable, but just so you get my point, here are a few of my favourites:

- Simply put, if you sleep well, you feel well and have energy to exercise and make healthy meals.

- Proper sleep helps blunt cortisol, which as we have learned, is a fat promoting, fat storing hormone.

- Sleep is a time for repair and regeneration. It is a time for your body to try and undo all the damage we have done through the day (which includes things like stress from hectic lifestyles, poor diet and sedentary lifestyles).

- Slumber provides an ideal time for our systems to detoxify. Think about it as a personalized nightly janitorial team.

- Sleep allows for the release of particular hormones like serotonin that make us feel good. Feeling more relaxed and happy allows us to utilize the bedroom for sex, which you will soon learn, is an important tool for stress management.

In addition to its wonderful sleep benefits, melatonin boots our energy levels, supports a healthy immune system, livens up our libido and supports muscle building and fat loss.

Since this chapter is on stress, I should also note that melatonin acts as a protection against the damaging effects of stress. Stress, as we have already learned, wreaks havoc on our system and is one of the main culprits of unfavourable weight gain.

GABA (Gamma-aminobutyric acid): This calming neurotransmitter is responsible for keeping the body relaxed, helping with digestion, sleep and preventing depression. Without enough GABA, factors like quality sleep and relaxation diminish our ability to make sound decisions and keep us happy. When these factors are compromised, it could be argued that healthy weight loss is much more difficult. In the journal of Molecular Brain Research, mice exposed to repeated swim stresses resulted in decreased GABA levels. This argues the point that high levels of stress decrease GABA and therefore, can alter our ability to achieve sustainable weight loss.

Thyroid hormones: This is a group of hormones that regulates your metabolism—also known as your ability to convert what you eat and drink into energy. If this isn't working optimally, what do you think happens to the foods and drink you consume? You guessed it—storage, not energy expenditure!

Glucagon: This fat-busting hormone signals our bodies to release stored sugar when we eat a balanced diet that is high enough in protein. Glucagon also fires when we exercise; in both instances, our blood sugars drop, glucagon is released and sugar is expended for energy. When our bodies are stressed, the delicate equilibrium of our blood sugars is disrupted and weight loss becomes more difficult to control, as glucagon is no longer functioning the way it should be to promote fat loss.

Progesterone: This is a key player in hormonal health. Progesterone helps to build bone density and supports libido. It plays a massive role in pregnancy by helping to make sure the mother's immune system does not attack a growing fetus.

Progesterone is a natural sleep aid and helps to lower blood pressure. When you're stressed, a deficiency in progesterone is created as your body steals it away from its normal functioning to help make cortisol.

Adrenalin: You know the moment when you slam the brakes on an icy patch of road and your heart takes a giant leap? That's adrenalin kicking into high gear. It's a stress hormone secreted in response to a perceived threat; in this case, an accident. Some symptoms you might have experienced include sweating, increased heart rate, trembling or shaking and dizziness.

In the right amounts, adrenalin can help promote fat loss. However, under chronic stressful conditions, constant adrenalin can wear you out! According to the Mayo Clinic, "the long-term activation of the stress-response system—and the subsequent overexposure to cortisol and other stress hormones—can disrupt almost all your body's processes. This puts you at increased risk of numerous health problems, including:

- Anxiety

- Depression

- Digestive problems

- Heart disease

- Sleep problems

- Weight gain

- Memory and concentration impairment"

Testosterone: Too little or too much of this masculinizing hormone can cause any woman to pack on the pounds. Low testosterone caused by the aging process or factors like stress and/or obesity can slow down our natural fat burning, while excess testosterone is often the result of overproduction by the adrenal glands (remember, these are our stress glands). The unfortunate consequence of having too much testosterone for women is often weight gain. According to Dr. Natasha Turner, author of The Hormone Diet, "The key to lowering testosterone is stress management (i.e. balancing cortisol) and controlling insulin levels…"

Growth hormone: This short-lived hormone is produced while we are in deep sleep. For those of you who wake periodically through the night, listen up! Growth hormone plays a major role in muscle growth and body fat percentage; the greater our muscle mass, ultimately, the lower our body fat will be. Sounds great, right? Right! So let's get you sleeping properly.

Why do we wake up in the night? There are numerous reasons people have trouble falling and/or staying asleep.

One of the first questions I ask clients is to rate their sleep on a scale of 1 to 10, where 10 represents you falling asleep well, staying asleep and waking feeling rested, and 0 is none of those things.

Sleep, as it turns out, is a problem for most of my clients. If you have no trouble sleeping consider yourself lucky.

In my practice, the most common sleep problems are the result of:

- Stress (thinking too much, hormonal imbalances caused by stress)

- Blood sugar imbalances caused by a high-carb diet and or infrequent eating patterns

- Eating/drinking too close to bedtime

Now it's your turn now to rate your sleep!

Circle the appropriate number based on your sleep

1	2	3	4	5	6	7	8	9	10

It's Just A Thought

You can see clearly from the evidence that stress can interfere with your ability to stay asleep. If you can't stay asleep, you won't produce growth hormone. And if you don't produce growth hormone, then how the heck can you stay hormonally balanced? If you're not balanced, then guess what? You store fat. It's as simple as that!

According to Dr. Mark Hyman, author of The Blood Sugar Solution, "Stress is a thought. That's it. No more, no less."

If this is true, why are so many of us dealing with chronic stress and all the health implications that come along with it, when stress is merely "just thoughts"?

There's no one answer to this. I personally believe it's our insane need to have the most, be the best, get the biggest, drive the fastest - mentality that keeps us stressed.

As a result of our constant thirst for more, we sleep less and eat out of convenience. If you look at our European neighbours, their lifestyles are much different. In many cases, physical possession isn't even important outside of necessities.

If we can agree that Dr. Hyman is onto something when he states that stress is merely a thought, then perhaps we can start digging deep and figure out what really is important.

Is staying up until 2 or 3 a.m. every night to get all those (let's face it) often unnecessary e-mails answered going to make you happier? Is getting angry with the driver in the next lane going to make you feel better?

While you work towards changing your outlook on the way you live your life, here are some other suggestions to make sure you're maximizing your efforts!

Tips For Dealing With Stress

"The most important weight loss muscle is the Brain. Change your Mind, Change your Body."

~Unknown

Sleep

Sleep is absolutely crucial for looking and feeling our best. The following are strategies I use, in addition to recommending a balanced diet and supporting stress levels, to help clients fall and stay asleep.

Falling asleep. I find one of the most beneficial tools for helping clients fall asleep faster is by developing sleep rituals. These are a set of habits that should be done nightly so that your sleep system has consistency and knows what to expect at this time of day. You can design your own sleep ritual, but keep in mind these key ideas:

Tip #1: Set the mood: Turn the lights down in your home so your natural sleep hormones can start kicking in. Use lamps and candles to provide low lighting in the later hours of the day. Avoid or limit super action-packed TV shows and movies that raise sleep-inhibiting hormones like adrenalin.

Tip #2: Have a tea break. There are so many wonderful products on the market these days that cater to sleep issues. One of my favourite suggestions is Sleepy Time Teas. Look for ingredients like passionflower, lemon balm and chamomile. Steep 1 bag into about ½ a mug of hot water. Not only will these herbs help relax your system but the tea itself provides a fat-fighting alternative to unnecessary snacking at night. Drink this about 45 minutes before you go to bed.

Tip #3: Warm up and cool down. Having a warm shower right before bed will inevitably result in a slight cooling of the body. It is actually at cooler temperatures that sleep is triggered, according to Dr. Natasha Turner. Just before bed, hop into the shower or bath for a quick rinse, just long enough to warm your body up.

Tip #4: Set a bedtime and stick to it. I believe that our bodies thrive on routine. Setting a schedule allows our systems to learn what to expect. Plan to get 7-8 hours of uninterrupted sleep per night. Move your schedule ahead by 15 minutes each night until you reach this goal.

With this said, getting to bed at the right times is also super imperative. I believe you will get a much better quality of sleep between the hours of 10 p.m. to 6 a.m. than you would if you slept from 1 a.m. to 9 a.m. This is largely due to hormonal rhythms.

Tip #5: Read. At the end of a long day, there is nothing more I look forward to than snuggling into bed with a good book.

In university, I struggled to stay awake and study from my textbooks as I always have associated reading with sleep.

Reading gives you a break from life stuff and gives you a calming escape. Sometimes on stressful days, I'll just pick up a book for 10 or 15 minutes and get away.

Reading also helps tire the eyes so it's a fantastic tool for helping people fall asleep quicker. Choose books that interest you but that don't keep you up until all hours of the night and set limits in case the book is hard to put down!

Tip #6: Guided calm. If ever I have a difficult time falling asleep than my go-to is a guided meditation. One of my favourite sites is www.calm.com (more about this to follow).

I remember when I bought my first house I was insanely excited and feel like I didn't sleep for a month! Had I known about guided meditations at this time I'm sure I would have gotten some zzzz's. Guided meditations help you focus on something other than what you are thinking or stressing about. They calm the mind and body, better allowing you to slip off into sleepyville.

Often people are skeptical about this type of suggestion. My tip to you is to be open to it and give it a shot before judging whether you are into this or not.

Tip #7: If you struggle to get your butt to bed, set an evening alarm that will go off LOUDLY for whatever time you want to be on your way there. The trick? You'll have to get upstairs to turn the alarm off—and then you'll stay there for bedtime.

Tip #8: Have sex! I couldn't end this section without touting the sleep-promoting benefits of a good romp. Not only is sex considered exercise (which is wonderful for burning calories, then falling and staying asleep, I might add), but according to WebMD.com and psychiatrist Sheenie Ambardar MD, "After orgasm, the hormone prolactin is released, which is responsible for the feelings of relaxation and sleepiness" after sex. So get to it—literally! Put this down and get busy!

Other rituals you can incorporate that might help with falling asleep:

- soft and calming music

- journaling

- aromatherapy

- hot tub or sauna

> *Nancy here: Family reading can be a part of your routine (the boys and I read in bed together nightly). I tuck them in, and then I stay upstairs to read my own book and go to bed. My chores are done both with my children and for the moment. I also wake up earlier than the kids so I have an hour in the morning, when my tank is full, to prep dinner for the next night, etc.*

Exercise

Whoever said that exercise is a great tool for stress relief is absolutely right! We know this, yet many don't fully understand exactly why exercise is so critical for our mental and emotional health.

Exercise helps stimulate serotonin; simply put, it makes you feel happier. When you feel happier, any clingy stressors don't seem as important.

Exercise helps reduce stress hormones. When I work out, I imagine those nasty, "I'm going to make you store fat," hormones fizzling away into thin air. This always makes me feel lighter!

It burns calories. Duh.

Great exercise options:

- Yoga

- Tai chi

- Strength training in a gym or in your home

- Tennis

- Brisk walking

- Join a boot camp

- Swimming

Whatever exercise you choose, good for you! Simply doing something is far better than doing nothing—the research proves it!

My personal tips to happy, sustaining exercise:

- Choose something you like. Why in the world would you stick to something if you hate it? I do not enjoy being in the gym. Instead, I run, walk, do strength training home videos and practice Pilates.

- Build it into your calendar. I schedule my workouts as I would a meeting. I plan the workouts weeks in advance so nothing gets in the way. If something comes up, then, oh well, but for the majority of the time I've committed myself to those blocks.

Limit allergenic foods

In addition to the mental, emotional stressors we have to deal with on a day-to-day basis, certain foods can also add stress to the body. Add these all up and sometimes it's just too much for our systems.

I'm sure you can guess what foods I'm referring to—typically white flours and sugars and highly processed foods that contain trans fats (reference the list from Chapter 4 of crap foods that you want to ditch).

However, for some people, seemingly healthy, everyday foods can also be stressful if you're sensitive or intolerant to the item. Examples of these foods include eggs, tomato, citrus, soy, dairy and certain grain varieties like wheat, rye, barley and spelt.

Whatever the reason for the sensitivity, prolonged consumption of ANY food that causes symptoms is toxic to the system and should be removed.

If offending foods are not removed, they then put a strain on the system (stressing it out) and, in turn, create inflammation. Inflammation, in the short term, is a normal and natural healing measure, but too much inflammation over too long of a time can create problems and can impede our ability to deal with stress properly.

Furthermore, prolonged exposure to any toxic food strains our immune systems, creating a whole new set of problems.

If you notice, after cleaning up your diet and practicing mindful eating habits, that any food creates uncomfortable gastro-intestinal symptoms, fatigue or rashes, consider removing that food for a period of about 30 days. If at this point, when you reintroduce the food, you notice symptoms that had disappeared come back, the best solution would be to eliminate this food for the time being to reduce stress on the body.

Anti-inflammatory foods

Just as important as it is to remove offending foods, it's equally important to provide high quality, anti-inflammatory foods to support the system. These include all those delicious, brightly coloured foods like blueberries, turmeric and kale!

Eating an abundance of these immune-supporting, brain-boosting, inflammation-fighting foods will not only make you feel energized and strong but will also work on those tiny cells of yours to unburden the system of unwanted junk that impede our ability to deal with other stressors that come our way.

Eating a minimum of two to three cups of veggies per day is a great start to meeting your quota of stress-supporting foods!

Meditation/breathing

If stress is just a series of thoughts, then it makes sense that calming the mind could calm the stress.

As a business owner, I have in the past—and sometimes still do—feel unequipped for the challenges I face.

As you could imagine, this would prove stressful to anyone… but especially to "A" type personalities like me. Over the years, and through trial and error, I have had to equip myself with tools for dealing with those challenges in a healthier way.

Breathing and meditation has become one of those tools for me.

The first time I was ever introduced to meditation was in nutrition school.

I did not bite. I thought it was silly and a useless waste of time (remember you are talking to a list-making, do-a-million-things-in-a-day, can-never-move-fast-enough, A-type gal).

Fast forward to now and I'm in. I have seen first-hand, people crippled by stress and anxiety calm their nerves with a few conscious moments of breathing—and that's all meditation is. Breathing or meditation, whatever you want to call it, is simply conscious presence. According to the meditation society, meditation is a "consciousness that brings serenity, clarity, and bliss. It is the awareness that arises from paying attention on purpose, in the present moment, non-judgmentally, to things as they are."

Consciousness or awareness is ultra-important for those who have a hard time shutting off their brains, or for those who tend to over think the stuff going on in their lives. Typically, it's this "stuff" that creates the stress.

If you are focusing on being more aware of the present moment, you won't be ruminating about the past or worrying about the future.

Bring conscious or mindful helps to increase awareness, disrupt automatic reactions, increase your ability to tolerate distressing emotions, and provide perspective.

Putting it into practice

The body-scan technique and the mindful eating exercise are two simple examples of mindful meditation practices that will get you started.

At the end of the chapter, I've also provided more resources, some of which I use myself. Remember there is no "right" and no "wrong" way to practice. The end goal is to calm the mind and achieve an overall greater sense of balance and contentment. Do what works and feels good to you.

#1 Mindful Eating Exercise

Begin the exercise by taking a food item (from your next meal) in the palm of your hand or set on the plate in front of you.

Imagine that you are a visitor from another universe. You've just landed on the planet and you've been given an object you're not familiar with. Your task is to gather as much information as you can about this object

1. Hold the food item in your hand and examine it.

2. Look closely at the item, observing details about its appearance. Notice the colour, feel the texture, weight and temperature and any other interesting characteristics. Imagine you have never seen this item before.

3. Now pick up the item and hold it close to your ear. Does it make a sound? If yes, is it high- or low-pitched? Loud or soft?

4. Bring the item close to your nose and carefully smell it. What do you notice? Is this a familiar smell to you? Is it a strong smell or one that can hardly be noticed? Take note of your body's reaction to this prolonged exposure to food although you haven't begun to eat it.

5. Now move the object over your lips and feel the texture as you move it along your lower and upper lips.

6. When you are ready, place the item in your mouth and run your tongue over it. Take notice of the flavours and textures as you explore the sensations in your mouth.

7. And now, moving the object over your teeth finally, take the object into your mouth and push it against the upper palate and lower palate, feeling every aspect of the object. Move the object between your teeth and slowly bite into it. Try to chew as slowly as possible. Notice the flavour that is in your mouth and pay attention to your body's reaction to the taste of the food item.

8. Work the item toward the back of the throat as you get ready to swallow it and then, swallow it. Observe its path as it travels down the throat and finally enters the stomach.

9. See what it feels like to be one object heavier, one object more energized, one object more powerful for being mindful of this process.

#2 The Body Scan Technique

Lie down on your back in a comfortable place, such as on a foam pad on the floor or your bed (but remember for this use, you are aiming to "fall awake" not fall asleep). Make sure that you will be warm enough. You might want to cover yourself with a blanket or do it in a sleeping bag if the room is cold.

Allow your eyes to gently close.

Feeling the rising and falling of your belly with each in breath and out breath.

Take a few moments to feel your body as a "whole" from your head to your toes, the envelope of your skin, the sensations associated with touch in the places you are in contact with the floor or bed.

Bring your attention to the toes of the left foot. As you direct your attention to them, see if you can direct or channel your breathing into your toes and out from your toes. It may take a while for you to get the hang of this. It may help to just imagine your breath traveling down the body from your nose into your lung and then continuing through the abdomen and down the left leg all the way to the toes and then back again and out through your nose.

Allow yourself to feel any and all sensations from your toes, perhaps distinguishing between them and watching the flux of sensations in this region. If you don't feel anything at the moment, that is fine too. Just allow yourself to feel *not just feeling anything.*

When you are ready to leave the toes and move on, take a deeper, more intentional breath in all the way down to the toes and, on the out breath, allow them to "dissolve" in your "mind's eye." Stay with your breathing for a few moments at least, and then move on to the sole of the foot, the heel, the top of the foot and then the ankle. Continue to breathe into and out from each region as you observe the sensations that you are experiencing, and then letting go of it and moving on.

Bring your mind back to the breath each time you notice that your attention has wandered off.

Continue to move slowly up your left leg and through the rest of your body as you maintain focus on the breath and on the feeling of the particular regions as you come to them, breathe with them, and let go of them.

Practice the body scan technique at least once a day.

Source ~ Jon Kabat Zinn, Ph.D

Supplementation

I find supplementing is often overlooked when it comes to dealing with stress. Although it should not be used exclusively for stress management, there is certainly a place for natural products in this conversation.

Below is a list of my five favourite natural supplements that can have beneficial effects on those dealing with stress and their most common effects on the body.

Remember that each person is unique and therefore, you'll need specific support to meet your individual needs. Make sure you consult your private healthcare practitioner before taking any product.

SUPPLEMENT	BENEFIT
RHODIOLA	- Reduces cortisol while uplifting mood and energy levels.
B-COMPLEX VITAMIN THAT INCLUDES INOSITOL	- B vitamins are depleted during stress so supplementing helps adrenals adapt - Inositol helps improve serotonin production (our happy chemical)
PASSIONFLOWER	- Sleep disruption is a common side effect of stress. This herb helps to relax the mind and body - Too little sleep can cause additional stress
VITAMIN C	- A potent antioxidant concentrated in our adrenal glands - Becomes depleted during stress - C helps keep our immune system strong and better able to cope during times of stress
TURMERIC	- A brightly coloured spice often used in Indian cooking. - Has potent anti-inflammatory properties to aid in management of stress and a variety of chronic conditions

Acupuncture

Acupuncture is an ancient healing technique used for the treatment of illnesses and diseases. This type of therapy goes back centuries. Today, if you scroll through scholarly articles on trials using acupuncture to help with any number of health concerns, you'll find plenty of information.

Luckily for us, acupuncture is used to relieve stress, too. According to the respected Cleveland Clinic, acupuncture "stimulates the body's ability to resist or overcome illnesses and conditions by correcting imbalances. Acupuncture also prompts the body to produce chemicals that decrease or eliminate painful sensations." The Journal of Autonomic Neuroscience: Basic and Clinical states that "acupuncture modulates endogenous regulatory systems, including the sympathetic nervous system, the endocrine system, and the neuroendocrine system".

In simple terms, this is basically saying that acupuncture has the ability to influence or control internal systems like hormones and the nervous system (which is partially controlled by the brain). We learned above that stress is a mental or emotional strain or tension, so it makes sense that acupuncture would be helpful!

There are many licensed acupuncturists out there. Make sure you find one that specializes in stress management acupuncture to ensure you are getting the best possible treatment for you.

Improving digestion

This is a pretty easy way of helping to support the body, not only in times of stress, but also in general.

We asked how often you get gassy, bloated or experience any gastrointestinal upset during the day or after eating in the quiz above. If this is something you experience, listen up! Symptoms like these after meals spell disaster for your immune system.

Think about it this way: if you are symptomatic after meals, a safe assumption is that you are not digesting food properly for one reason or another (and trust me, there are many reasons). If your body isn't breaking down fats, proteins, carbs and micro nutrients, then you're also not going to be absorbing and benefitting from these vital nutrients.

When this happens, your immune system can become compromised. Stress beats up your immune system—couple that with a lack of nutrients to support healthy immunity and your body will wear down faster than your stress-free, optimally digesting counterpart.

So what to do?

Chew your food, for Pete's sake!

Most people that walk into my practice smirk when we have "the digestion conversation" because they are fully aware that they barely take a breath between bites. It's no surprise to me that most people race through their meals; we are busy and we have too much on our plates (literally and figuratively). In general, we look at meals as more of an inconvenience than a time of fuel and enjoyment. So, aim to chew your food to a paste. Sounds gross maybe, but so does those whole chunks of undigested food that are landing in your intestinal system and putrefying. Do it.

Avoid liquids with your meals. Yep. Water and milk and juice and here it goes… yes, I'm going to go there… wine.

ALL liquids! Drinking fluids with your meals dilutes and washes away all those valuable digestive enzymes your body has worked so hard to make. Consider this: when you're stressed, your body lacks the ability to manufacture digestive enzymes optimally. Pair that with the fact you are washing these little guys away and no wonder you are gassing your husband out of the room after your meals!

For those of you who worry about taking medications or supplements or who want to enjoy small amounts of wine here and there, sip at only a ¼ cup of whatever you want. Doing so helps preserve your enzyme concentration and ensures your pipes are working!

Ctrl/Alt/Delete Negativity

Everything we think is our truth. "Every thought we think is creating our future."

My belief is that what we think shapes the direction we're headed. If stress is just a series of thoughts and those negative thoughts consume us and affect our body, then those thoughts are essentially worthless.

And if we continue to have these negative thoughts, we soon LEARN to have these thoughts and essentially default or (autopilot) to thinking the stressful thoughts.

Deep, huh?

Our brains are essentially like computers; the outcome of certain actions can be programmed in. If you hit "Ctrl/Alt/Delete" on your computer, you'll shut down the program you're running. So let's "Ctrl/Alt/Delete" our negative thoughts and perhaps the stress (and its effects) will be less severe.

How, you ask?

Many of my clients walk in my door stressed—granted, most don't know it at the time. Let's finally start to deal with the issues (stressors) that get in the way of weight loss success!

I use and recommend the following two techniques to help change the way I view my "stuff."

Change your point of view. You've heard the saying: "Are you a glass-half-empty type of person or a glass-half-full type of person?" Although it's cliché, I feel there is a lot of value in this question.

If every thought you have is tainted with negativity, do you not think this is stressful for your body?

Research is proving that the thoughts we have affect our body. For example, often when a person is under high stress, they get sick (we all know of that girl or guy who stresses about getting organized all week long before a sunny vacation and then the day after arriving, they come down with a cold… bummer!).

It's time to start being more conscious about the thoughts we have. I truly believe there is something good—or a valuable lesson to be found—in any lousy situation. We might need to dig pretty deep to find it, but it's there. Finding it will take the heaviness down a notch out of the seemingly negative situation.

For me, driving has always been a challenge. I suffered from classic road rage. If I got cut off, I went into a tizzy: my blood would boil, I'd mutter curse words under my breath and continue on in anger. It wasn't until many years of speaking to others about their stress that I realized this was a problem.

Now, when I get cut off, my thoughts automatically shift gears (no pun intended). I think to myself: "That man or women must be on their way to the hospital because someone they love has had an emergency!"

To me, that person almost has the right to cut me off; clearly their situation is far more important than me getting wherever I'm going. Of course, I know deep down they're likely not headed to the hospital, but thinking this way sure does diffuse the situation in the moment and makes me feel better.

Distraction is another amazing technique I encourage everyone to utilize. Sure, you can find a positive twist on any situation, but sometimes that just isn't going to cut it. Sometimes we need to drop the thought and move on. Why continually mull it over, rehash the conversation or worry what you could have done differently? The truth is, stressing about it will just contribute to the waistline you are already unhappy with. Distraction is simple. Here's how:

- Acknowledge your thought

- Decide to think about something else, like your upcoming vacation or the next healthy meal you're planning... or sing a song you like!

Consciously stopping the negative thoughts or finding a positive spin gives you the ability to "Ctrl/Alt/Delete" the "stuff." It takes time and energy, but eventually you'll notice you're more able to gravitate towards the positive and/or turn off the stuff that brings you down and contributes to your weight.

Finding Joy

What does joy look like to you? By definition, joy is "to experience great pleasure or delight." The simple act of doing something you love helps decrease cortisol as your brain gets redirected to things other than stress.

Research shows that pleasurable things like relaxing in the sun and getting a massage also help to raise serotonin levels, which we know is your "happy" hormone. So decide now what brings you joy and write them down.

Once you've identified the people and things that bring you joy, consider, when you feel stressed, reaching out to these people or activities to blunt the negativity.

Record here at least two people and two things or activities that bring you joy. If you have more than two each, great!

_____

_____

_____

You can find this exercise in the workbook!

=>> http://bonus.weightlossgspot.com

Sex

More and more research is supporting the fact that sex can have huge benefits on our health. It's been touted for its ability to lower blood pressure, strengthen our cardiovascular system, prevent certain cancers, as well as lower cortisol levels.

And it's no secret that stress impacts your libido. It simply sucks the fun out of sex!

Foods that replenish and soothe

Often we turn to ice cream, chips and wine as comfort food during times of stress. Although these provide instant gratification, eventually the guilt sets in and most of us end up feeling even worse.

The thing we need to remember in this situation is that stress is essentially in our heads, so knowing the facts and what to do about it allows us to get out of our own heads and take action on an unpleasant thought.

Now, I get it, a great glass of red after a hard day certainly helps, but making this a habit will, for many, ultimately lead to weight gain and additional stress. So in addition to the above strategies, consider the following foods for their healthy stress-busting properties.

- During times of stress, the body loses its stores of vitamin C from the adrenal glands. Kiwi, collard greens, red bell peppers, mustard and turnip greens are all rich in vitamin C and will help replenish what has been lost.

- Guacamole, nuts, asparagus and seafood are loaded with B vitamins, which as we have learned, are essential to healthy adrenal gland function.

- Spinach, raw chocolate and bananas are rich in magnesium, a mineral that helps regulate our cortisol levels and relax the body.

- Fresh water fish like salmon, trout and cod contain omega 3 fatty acids, which protect the heart from surges in stress hormones.

Hippocrates had it right when he said, "Let food be thy medicine and medicine be thy food." Let's use his thinking to find our Weight Loss G-Spot and start healing our bodies!

Alternative techniques

If the above tools and techniques do not resonate with you and/or you're looking for more options, here's a list of other stress management tools for you to research.

- The Emotional Freedom Technique (tapping technique) is a psychological acupressure technique that uses energy meridians in the body, similar to those used in acupuncture to treat physical and emotional ailments.

- Essential oils like orange and lavender are soothing to the nervous system

- Speak with a social worker or psychologist

- Affirmations

- Regular massage therapy

Okay. You've rated your stress level, taken a quiz and learned how to change how stress is impacting you. Now, summarize THREE things you are going to do differently, starting today (record BOTH what you're going to do and HOW you're going to do it.)

_____

_____

_____

At the beginning of this chapter, you took a mini-quiz that touched upon a few of the most common symptoms of chronic stress.

If you scored a number greater than five, consider that you might be in need of some stress support (see the above suggestions).

Whether you acknowledge this stress at this exact moment, I encourage to keep your test score in mind and look at how you behave and react a little more mindfully going forward. If and when you decide you need some guidance or support, send Nancy or I a note because we'd love to be a part of your journey! XO

michelle@strongnutritionandweightloss.com

Nancy@nancymilton.ca

> **Chapter 10: Keys to G**
>
> • Stress affects everyone differently; don't compare yourself against your neighbour.
>
> • Consider the symptoms in the quiz; if you experience more than five of these, perhaps you need to take a closer look at your stress and question whether this might be the culprit to your stubborn excess fat or your inability to lose weight.
>
> • There are sooooooo many things you can do to deal with your stress levels! You just have to be willing to try new things and get out of your comfort zone. Give it a chance... you might realize you're more comfortable (and relaxed) in the end.

Additional Helpful Resources

Books:

Transforming Stress, by Doc Childre

The Four Agreements, by Don Miguel Ruiz

Audio:

Calm.com

Eli Bay guided meditations (elibay.com)

FREE BOOK UPDATES, VIDEOS AND RESOURCES

Want to learn more? We have created a free workbook to go along with this book. You will also find a list of great documentaries, books, websites and other valuable bonus resources to will help you dive deeper!

Get access to your free bonus resources at http://bonus.weightlossgspot.com/

11

SHOE AND PENIS SIZE ARE CORRELATED... AND MORE MISCONCEPTIONS

Hi, Michelle back again! Here's my take on some of the big myths out there that might have you stumbling to know what is fact or fiction.

Does eating fat make me fat?

Do I have to give up all carbs to lose weight?

Will I have to spend all my time in the kitchen in order to be healthy?

These are not uncommon questions. It seems like these myths or misconceptions have been so ground into our heads by genius marketing initiatives and we're so easily influenced by those, "Well, I've heard_____"-type conversations.

As you read though this book, I'm assuming some of those same questions might enter your head. So, let's spend some time discerning myth from truth so you have what is, in my opinion, the most current information you need in order to attain your fat loss and health goals.

The Myth: High fat makes you fat.

The Truth: There are two camps still hashing out this argument. I know from my studies and through my experience that fat is good, but, of course, it depends on the type of fat we're talking about.

In Chapter 5, we learned about what fats are good for us and what fats you need to ban from your kitchen altogether. In essence, healthy fat provides energy, satiety and stability for our blood sugars and hormones, which is essential for healthy fat loss.

Can you eat too much of this good stuff? Definitely! But aiming for 4 to 5 servings of healthy fats per day (see Chapter 7 for explanations of serving sizes) will keep you in fat-burning mode.

The Myth: Being healthy is too hard.

The Truth: I always tell clients that the weight loss process, or simply improving your healthy lifestyle, is equally about what's in your head as what is in your mouth.

At the beginning, lifestyle changes can seem daunting and sometimes require more effort. Knowing this: it's all a state of mind! You can make this process as easy or difficult as you want with what you tell yourself. If you constantly begrudge the process and complain about it, than it will be hard and time consuming. Once you can commit, make peace with what is ultimately your own decision to change for the better, it becomes an extremely fulfilling experience that you'll want to continue with.

The Myth: You'll never eat junk food again.

The Truth: I know that running out for fast food is way easier than preparing a meal after a long day, I also know that parties and barbecues present sometimes irresistible temptations that make you feel like a failure if you indulge.

Living a healthier lifestyle doesn't mean that these things are necessarily off the table. Consider the 80:20 rule; if 80 percent of your choices are clean, low sugar, nutrient-dense foods, then you are hitting the mark!

I'm often asked, "Do you ever eat anything unhealthy?" The answer is YES! I love chocolate and the occasional indulgence. The difference between me and many others is that I limit treats to occasions when I'm in a social setting or special events like birthdays and holidays - this way it feels more like a treat than a regular part of my diet.

> *Nancy here: Let's be clear. You're transitioning to eating more like Michelle. She's comfortably at the weight she enjoys and this is her lifestyle. She has a lovely balance going on. You can have it, too. Choices, people! Choices!*

Keep these tips in mind when making your "to eat or not to eat" decision:

Tip #1: Pick your poison! If you don't 100 percent LOVE that treat, why eat it? Why not save your indulgence for a time where you will enjoy the treat so much more?

Tip #2: Is the treat worth the calories? If I answer no to this question, then skipping that "food" is a no-brainer!

Tip #3: Does this "food" or treat propel you toward your goal or away from your goal? If the answer is away, then perhaps going back to tip #2 and re-examining your decision would be wise.

The Myth: I must always buy organic.

The Truth: There are a lot of skeptics out there arguing that organic food isn't necessarily as organic or healthy as it's said to be. So considering its higher price point here's my take—if you can afford it, put your money where your mouth is—literally. At the very least, organic food has not been sprayed with chemical fertilizers, herbicides, pesticides or altered as a genetically modified organism. In the case of animals, organic meats are not pumped with antibiotics, growth hormones and are fed grains free of the above additives found in many traditional feeds.

If you can't afford all organic, consider buying organic for the foods you consume the most often or the foods that you can't peel or are more difficult to wash thoroughly, like broccoli and raspberries.

Consider making the organic choice on foods from the Dirty Dozen list in Chapter 4. These are the 12 foods that are said to be the most highly sprayed. This is an easy place to start and will not significantly increase your grocery bill.

The Myth: Being healthy is too time-consuming.

The Truth: I can't tell a lie. Living a healthy lifestyle does take a little more time, but I will argue that the benefits far outweigh the extra time spent to ensure you and your family are well cared-for. In my opinion, it's all about allotment of time. You can choose to spend the time sitting on the couch or you could take 15 minutes to do a little prep work for the next day. It's all a choice in the end!

Nancy here: Are you kidding me? If you've been following the chapters, you've already claimed back ¼ of your time because you're sleeping better, you're more energized and organized PLUS, you have clear goals. Suck it up, buttercup! YOU are worth this.

Consider the following tips to make being healthy less of an inconvenience and more just a part of who you are and what you do.

- Plan ahead. Each week, my husband and I sit down and plan out what each dinner will look like. Doing this allows me to buy enough groceries for the entire week (eliminating the need to make several trips to the store).

  Nancy here: See, Michelle just granted you more of your time back! You now only need to grocery shop once a week.

  This also takes the guesswork out of deciding what's for dinner after a long day. If the plan is to have glazed salmon with sweet potato and rapini on Wednesday, that's what I'll make—no need to hem, haw and waste valuable time trying to brainstorm.

- Consider making four weeks of menus and reusing them for a few months. If you create four weeks of meals, you won't eat the same meal more than once every month. Brilliant, right?

- Make extra! Whatever you eat for dinner can easily be packed up for lunch the next day. Again, this not only eliminates time spent thinking and then prepping lunches, it will save you from having to go buy a meal that most likely won't be as healthy.

- Prep to your heart's content. I get some pushback from clients on this suggestion, but think of it this way: prepping allows you to make bulk meals in your free time that will support your meals and snacks during the week. Making a hearty soup can act as a side dish, whole meal or snack. The time it takes you to make this on the weekend will save so much time and frustration than if you had to think of, prep and pack a new meal and/or snack daily during your busy week.

The Myth: Weight loss is simply a factor of calories in versus calories out.

The Truth: Unfortunately, thinking about weight loss in these terms isn't this simple. Think about it this way: a 500 calorie meal comprised of chicken, vegetables and sweet potato, and a 500 calorie meal consisting of a Big Mac and fries are very different in terms of their nutritional value, yet they have similar calorie counts.

If this theory that weight loss is simply a factor of calories in versus calories out were correct, than eating either meal would allow you to maintain a good health status and lose weight successfully. But we all know that eating fast food can lead to weight gain, higher cholesterol levels, low energy, etc. If you don't believe me, watch the movie Supersize Me.

Despite the similarities in calorie count, it's what that calorie is comprised of that makes all the difference. A calorie that is made up of poor quality meats, sugar, white processed flours and trans fats is going to affect the body much differently than a calorie made up of lean protein, vitamins, healthy fats, fibre-rich vegetables and energy-packed complex carbohydrates.

Knowing that the quality of calorie will affect our body in different ways, we can also easily conclude that our ability to burn that calorie off and lose weight will be different based also on the quality consumed.

The Myth: If it's low in calories, it's a healthy food.

The Truth: When it comes to labelling on packages, we often don't focus enough on the nutritional facts, and in my opinion, these are super important. A calorie, according to Merriam-Webster, is merely a measurement of "heat to indicate the amount of energy that foods will produce in the human body," and while this is important, most of us do not recognize the importance of other items on a nutritional label, like sugar and the ingredients list.

We learned in Chapter 5 that sugar is added to far too many products to make them more palatable. Sugar disrupts the immune system, makes us crave more sugar and leads to weight gain.

Ingredients in packaged products can be varied and misleading. You'll find everything from artificial sweeteners and colours, preservatives, trans fatty acids, thickeners, emulsifiers and so much more! Buyer beware, sometime the calorie (as we learned in Chapter 4) is only one part of the puzzle.

The Myth: You need to be a vegetarian to be healthy.

The Truth: In my clinical experience, I have witnessed that many vegetarians aren't eating a balanced diet. The emphasis on grain products is far too high and while vegetables are typically adequate, proteins are often lacking.

The problem with this lies in the fact that proteins are one of the most vital components of a healthy diet. As we learned already, proteins are one of the building blocks of the body. They're the heal and repair macronutrient. When the goal is weight loss, it's difficult to lose weight and maintain muscle mass without consuming enough protein.

If your choice is vegetarianism, this is perfectly fine; just ensure your diet is balanced with the correct amount of fats, proteins and carbohydrates. If you need help, let me know!

The Myth: You must avoid carbs to lose weight.

The Truth: Remember from earlier discussions that the word "carbohydrate" is an umbrella term for many different healthy food groups, including vegetables, fruits, legumes, dairy products, root vegetables and grains like rice and quinoa.

I'm very conscious that you take this away from this discussion: I am NOT reducing your carbohydrate consumption. I am merely limiting your grain consumption.

Carbs, specifically complex carbs, are energy-packed nutrients that provide us an array of health benefits. Eating these foods are important for balanced health. Providing you eat the proper balance and keep grains limited, weight loss is entirely possible!

The Myth: Everyone should eat gluten free.

The Truth: It seems that going gluten free has become somewhat fashionable and more and more people are hopping on this bandwagon. Reducing overall gluten and wheat intake from your diet is a viable option that could help support healthy fat loss; for most people though, weight loss isn't dependent solely upon eating this way. Whatever your personal decision is, own it!

Let's highlight the pros and cons of this type of lifestyle:

Pros

- Gluten and wheat products are often genetically modified and therefore, more difficult for our bodies to digest and then absorb nutrients. Removing these products from our diet takes stress away from these systems and allows for better overall digestive capabilities. Gluten free grains include (but not limited to) quinoa, rice and uncontaminated oatmeal.

- Eliminating wheat and gluten from our diets by default also reduces or removes unnecessary snacking on junk foods. Many people lose some weight without even trying because they're unable to mindlessly snack or overindulge at parties and gatherings.

Cons

- Gluten free products are often higher in sugar

- Gluten free products often tend to be produced with white grains like white rice and potato flour. These are higher on the glycemic index; eating them will spike your blood sugars (remind yourself of the cookie plunge from Chapter 4).

The Myth: Healthy food costs too much.

The Truth: In a way, this is correct. The first grocery store trip to stock up on new, healthier options can be a bit pricier.

After this trip, I would argue that it's all about what you buy and when. Here are some tips for keeping your kitchen stocked with healthy options while on a budget.

- Buy seasonal. In-season food has travelled a shorter distance and therefore, it will generally cost less (it's also fresher!).

- Don't buy all organic. Maybe this isn't the right option for you yet. Work your way towards this slowly if you want.

- Be flexible. Even though you always buy X type of apple doesn't mean you can't sub that out for the variety that's on sale that day; try not to be as rigid in your purchases!

  Nancy here: In my opinion, the Honey Crisp Apple is the Queen of the Apple Kingdom. It's easy for me to reach for one of these beauties for a snack, versus "Ugh, I don't want an apple!" Yes, this kind costs more but guess what? I'll eat them versus let them rot in my fridge.

- Plan your weekly meals to avoid waste. Your weekly grocery list will highlight everything you NEED and helps with reducing impulse purchases. Doing this also ensures that you have what you need and that fresh foods will not end up in your compost bin.

- Buy food in bulk. Bulk stores are great as they eliminate the packaging process; often the piece of the puzzle that costs a lot of money. Consider buying your nuts, seeds, legumes, spices, nut butters, etc. there to keeps costs lower.

- Also think about preparing your foods in bulk. Soups, stews and chili are fabulous options that take very little time or money to prepare, but last for many meals.

- Use leftovers. Try to find interesting ways to use leftover foods. Chicken, rice and veggies one night can be turned into fajitas the next night!

- Grow your own food! Why not start a small family garden? This will cost less than buying these same items, plus it's super satisfying watching foods grow that you've put your love and care into. And then you get to eat them!

- Check flyers. Apps like Checkout51, which notifies you of price breaks, are available for your Smartphone. Use your resources, people!

The Myth: Low fat = low fat.

The Truth: Repeat after me, low fat foods will not reduce your belly fat! Say that over and over until you start believing it! The truth it, low fat foods are typically higher in sugar than their regular fat counterparts. Food manufacturers add in sweetness to low fat foods to make them more palatable. Fat = taste. Once the taste is gone, so are many consumers.

The other problem with low fat foods—we assume, because they are low fat, we can eat more.

Think about this: at Halloween, we'll pop a few of those mini chocolate bars into our mouths without batting an eye.

But, many of us would hesitate or feel really guilty about eating a whole chocolate bar in that same time. What gives? You probably ate more of the little ones than you wanted to, but because they're small and cute and "only 100 calories" it doesn't seem like a big deal. The point here—don't reach for fat-free options in the hope you can eat more of them.

When picking foods at the store, try avoiding the low fat options over their full fat neighbours. Of course, this isn't a hard and fast rule because it depends on what foods we're speaking about, but in general, if it's a whole food, take the fat and skip the sugar! Remember we're supposed to have some fats in our diet—not white, processed sugar.

The Myth: Detoxing is the best way to clean out your body.

The Truth: If you are following the plan, by cleaning up your diet and lifestyle, getting more sleep, water and exercise and if you're reducing stress and finding more overall joy. Bravo! You are in fact detoxifying your body!

Once you have done these things and if next steps need to be taken, or if stubborn fat is hanging on, connect with a qualified professional (ME!) and we can move into a more advanced detoxification program that your body can handle.

I hope this has helped debunk some myths for you. Now that you have a plan you're following, and have answers to those pressing questions, it's time to own it!

Chapter 11: Keys to G

- Don't assume just because it's all the rage or a popular belief that it is true. Get the facts.

- We all have perspectives on things. Time to shift your myths to better your life—your healthier life!

12

I'M GOING TO...

Nancy here: Let's talk about taking ownership of your G-Spot!

What music plays in your head when the pressure's on?

When you know that you have to deliver—or else?

CUE THAT MUSIC!

This whole chapter—every single word—is about ownership. Throughout this book, we've spoken repeatedly about owning it. It's really a different way to say ownership and in our opinion, sounds less corporate.

And yes! "Own it IN YOUR SOUL" is a favourite saying of mine and I can proudly share that a client has actually embossed it on a shirt for me! I LOVE IT!

So, here's to you OWNING it. Let's get clear on what looks like.

When I meet with any new coaching client, we clearly define parameters for each other. Through my coach training, the term I learned for this is "Designing an Alliance."

This defines what they will need from me and what I will need from them to make our coaching relationship work—AND get results.

287

Having a thorough conversation gives us each clarity of roles, wants and how to get there as effectively as possible.

I actually practice this Designing an Alliance ritual in all aspects of my life: in my friendships, family-ships and biz-ships. As a result, I have the easiest break-ups ever! Why, you ask? Because we're both clear on what we need from each other to make it work, and when it's not, we can clearly see the miss, and either make a change or exit.

Here's the catch: I'm one of two authors of this book. You and I are now connected—but how will you hold yourself to your end of the bargain?

Here's my experience on this. When you are working with someone with mutual goals or interests and you're working on a project together, this, of course, seems straightforward and smart.

But what do you do when you have different goals (i.e. trying to understand someone you share children with, but live under two roofs with two very different parenting styles)? Or what if you're working independently and need to hold yourself accountable?

An alliance has to go two ways to support accountability and consequences. Specific to your weight loss goals, you want to have an alliance with someone who is mutually interested and will call you out if you step over the parameter line. Because let's be clear: few can hold themselves accountable; isn't that why you're in this situation?

In the case of you, us and this book, how will we know if you are consistently doing what you said you'd do? You need to come up with parameters for yourself.

Hope Is Not A Strategy!

As you know from other hope attempts (like winning the lottery), it can only get you so far. You need to consider and record what you need to do to hold yourself accountable. These parameters (or standards) are to take care of you, to ensure that you stay consistent, objective, and rational when dealing with someone (a person that may cause friction, which drives you to a quick food fix) or something (like a buffet!)

Basically, it's GO time and it's up to you. All of it! Everyone has choices to make. Some choices are much easier than others. Getting clear on your parameters, then holding yourself to those parameters, allows you to own it.

It's important you have personal parameters specific to this weight loss journey because:

- You're changing things in your life (for the better) and with parameters they are easier to follow through on.

- Clarity of your parameters on HOW to maintain your new health is like having instructions and ingredients for a recipe you've never made, or directions to a place a few hours away that you've never been to. Parameters are your Platinum Plan!

- It's the consistent reminder that you are the priority. Somehow you forgot that.

Having intentions is key to success in anything. Your parameters clearly hold your intentions in check.

It's time. You are twelve chapters in!

You've considered, written, envisioned, cleaned cupboards, shopped, worked hard and released emotions. Good on you! All that effort could stop here—or you can own it.

Our vote? OWN IT!

Here are my parameters to my G-Spot of Weight Loss:

- I grocery shop weekly using shopping lists based on specific recipes I've planned ahead of time for the week that I am really looking forward to eating.

- My home is completely refined sugar-free. Period. There is no flexibility here.

- My vision board is portable. It travels with me wherever I may be so I can start each day clear on my intention. Every morning starts with my intention.

- *"I am healthy, in control, love myself, and I am my priority."* I start each day stating this. I sometimes add more to it. I say it to myself in the day when I need to hear it. Sometimes I hear it a couple times in an hour.

- I have five (human, individual) touchstones. I rotate my touchstones weekly. Every week I reach to one of the five touchstones (people I support, who support me) to update them on where I am with my parameters.

- I write down what I eat every day and have someone waiting to receive it daily. If they don't, they call me. I, too, need help with accountability.

- I know who to call or contact when I can't shake the "I'm stuck in the missionary position" feeling.

  Michelle here: For me, parameters or consistencies are super important to keep me level. I thrive on having a plan to keep me on track and in line with my health goals.

The big one for me is thinking ahead. If I can plan out a week of meals, I won't get caught in the cookie jar because I'm starving and without a plan!

I share these with you as a starting point. Each of us has unique needs, qualities and expectations.

If you didn't know yourself before you read this book, you sure as heck do now. Be clear, really clear on what parameters you must hold yourself to every day to stick this for good. List those parameters. Be specific.

MY PARAMETERS to OWNing my Life (remember to write these in your workbook)

_____

_____

_____

Ta-da!

Your parameter list is complete. Now, what are you going to do with it?

Throughout this book, you've uncovered and learned about yourself.

This process has given you insight specific to how you get things done and what you need to keep yourself motivated. Consider these discoveries when deciding how to use your parameter list.

My list is written on a large post-it note and it resides on my bathroom mirror. And because sometimes when I'm away from home, it feels harder to stick to parameters, I have a second list, which includes my daily intentions, folded up in my wallet and easily accessible.

Mull over how you've done things in the past. This reflection needs to include those times you were successful as well as the times you weren't.

When you were rewarded with a win, think about what got you there, from a tricks and techniques standpoint? What made it difficult for you? Your new approach needs to be easy and reinforced daily. Decide how you will use your parameters to STAY successful.

Earlier, I acknowledged that I choose five people (I call them my touchstones) to support me, within my parameters, in my journey.

Let me bottom-line this for you: I have made the challenge of losing weight the hardest thing ever in my life, and I've spent over 20 years doing so. Knowing this, how foolish would I be to not set myself up with the support needed to continue my success and to cherish it as a life priority? FOOLISH.

I chose my touchstones based on my personal needs and the areas I find hardest to commit to.

Specific to me, here's my list of what I need from my touchstones:

- I continue to record what I am eating daily and forward it to my support system(s) for review and feedback.

- Writing down my intake is always something I have loathed, so my goal, as I continue to be successful and my healthy habits get more deeply ingrained, is to move to weekly recording submissions.

- A weigh-in challenge. I don't own a scale, but I meet a friend each week for a close-to-naked morning weigh-in. The partner aspect keeps us both in check. Our weight is charted. We then revise our plan for the week based on the number, our stress levels, measurements and how we feel, etc.

- I have some friends that consider their kitchen a playground. They can't wait to get in there, enjoy themselves and be creative. For me, the kitchen is like a forest fire—I grab what I need and get out as fast as I can! Understanding that I'm still mastering what playing in my kitchen looks like, I have two kitchen playground friends I rely on to provide EASY, reliable recipes when I'm feeling blah with my meals.

This is my team!

Experts: Depending on my mental strength and the time of year, I have a variety of people to plug into for accountability and motivation. My team includes a nutritionist and naturopath for their knowledge and different perspective on my progress and an Activity Organizer, a friend who never stops researching the next fun goal for us to master and keeps me solid on my workout regime. I have a tennis coach, a group tennis clinic, a boot camp and a yoga studio- all of which I have signed up for and they, the instructors, also watch for consistent participation.

The You-Get-Me Touchstone: Name the emotion and I can share it with this person. There's no judgement, no answers, no problem solving. I receive love, listening, and support… lucky me!

Your turn. You know yourself.

What kind of support do you need and how will you receive it? Be really clear on both points. GO.

_____

_____

_____

Next? Consequences.

Although I've been impacted by consequences in my life, my awareness of creating them for myself didn't resonate until I completed my coaching training.

It's important for me to actually clarify what my consequence will be if I don't do (or own) what I said I would do. From the get go, I've already established what my pain point will be.

Let me describe this in a different way.

As we shared earlier, the fact is, 77 percent of people break their New Year's resolutions.

My guess is that this isn't a crazy surprise to you, but you might not have thought the number of resolution casualties would be so high.

There are a variety of reasons for the miss: these include too-lofty goals, a lack of game plan to get results, low motivation, little follow-up or attention to consequences. Knowing we've spoken about the majority of these already, it's time to talk consequences.

What does the word consequence mean to you?

Consequence is commonly described as the default to an incomplete action.

Ironically, the word consequence specific to this book, and to weight loss, is all about lack of action. Our ask of you, and therefore, your ask to yourself is: "What will my consequence be if I don't do this?"

Often times, we consider the reverse: "What will I get if I do this?" We focus on the reward. There is merit in focusing on the reward; however, we feel you need to be just as clear with what happens if you don't do it.

If we focus only on the reward, we never know what we don't have.

Remember what we learned in Chapter 2? If the reward seems too lofty, it can be easily pushed aside. Make it believable and achievable!

Visualizing a consequence for not following through gives us the reality of the situation, a reality we sometimes avoid or are even oblivious to.

With coaching, there's always homework for my clients. The client creates what the homework is and the completion date. My next question is always along the lines of, "And what will the consequence be if you don't?"

This is one of the reasons people look for coaches. We help them get clear on what they want and holding themselves to making it happen. My clients quickly learn about creating and holding themselves to consequences. They deserve results. And so do you.

Over the years, I've heard the whole gamut of consequences.

Here are some examples:

If I don't _____ by _____, I will:

- Lose my morning coffee

- Pay double for my next coaching session

- Lose my Saturday treat

- Work out for three extra hours this week

Whatever consequence is created, it needs to resonate with you in such a way that it holds you to completing what's important to you. Pause now, and draft five potential consequences for yourself. Remember, they need to light a fire under your butt!

1._____

2._____

3._____

4._____

5._____

Review the list you've just completed. Circle the two consequences you dread most, the two that will challenge you, the two that make you gulp like something big and important is at stake.

This is your starting point.

Now, who are you reporting to? It needs to be someone who won't let you off the hook or take pity on you.

_____

_____

_____

You can find this exercise in the workbook!

=>> http://bonus.weightlossgspot.com

What mechanism will you put in place with the above person for follow-up?

Here's a personal example. For the first month of my accountability, I email a girlfriend every night before bed with a report of three things: one thing that I did well during my day that I would repeat the next day, one thing I'd stop doing and one thing I'd start doing. At the end of the first month, this routine moved to once a week.

How will they trust that you will report in completely and honestly?

Real-life example: I'm playing this role for two clients right now. One of the two clients emails me once a day at 3 p.m. with one statement that holds her accountable. The other client has 24 hours to contact me if she has strayed from her plan.

How will you be held accountable? Be specific.

_____

_____

_____

Taking it up a notch, consider how you will practice holding yourself accountable and executing your own consequences (or rewarding yourself).

Once you learn how to do this, in our opinion, you can learn how to do anything!

What will I do to help me hold myself to my actions?

Some of my personal examples include: waking 30 minutes earlier than usual to set my intentions for the day and meditation. Preparing a great afternoon snack to look forward to because that's a hard time of day for me, food journaling after every food encounter and catching where I'm at in that moment is how I hold myself accountable.

This chapter is geared towards arming yourself with key tools to keep you accountable to this process and your goal. But at the end of the day, you need to want this and you need to execute the plan. The title of this chapter is "I'm Going To"… so tell us, tell yourself, tell a friend what and how you are going to do what you need to do in order to succeed. Whatever the plan is, do it again and again and again until you have it down pat and have truly found Your Weight Loss G-Spot.

Chapter 12: Keys to G

- Owning this process, your weight loss process is paramount; hope is not a strategy.

- Make a plan, have someone help cheer you on and keep you accountable until this stuff becomes your life.

- Ensure you also have a plan or consequence to remind you about what is on the line.

- Connecting with your plan emotionally/passionately is key to sticking to it.

- You got this!

13

HOW TO MAKE IT A MULTIPLE

It's Michelle, standing by your finish line.

According to the Oxford Dictionary, the definition of a journey is "travelling from one place to another."

You should be proud, excited, elated—and maybe relieved—that you have conquered this part of your journey. Know there is more to come, but you have tackled the most challenging parts… and hopefully, overcome them!

Please take a giant breath and let this journey sink in. What a ride it was!

SO what's next?

If you haven't lost what you set out to lose from your original goal, then it's time to take stock of where you are, figure out how much more you want to lose and set yourself up with a new game plan. Our suggestion is to head back to Chapter 4 and make a new SMART plan based on your new set of goals. Remember to be specific and to reward yourself along the way.

If sabotaging foods are sneaking back into your fridge and pantry, clear them again and rid yourself of those pesky temptations. You'll find your instructions for this in Chapter 4.

Having an unscheduled cheat day happens to everyone. Get up, dust off that guilt and move on! What other choice do you have? I'm a nutritionist and I sometimes get off track. The important thing is to focus on what's important as soon as possible.

This would also be a good time to step on the scale again, take your measurements and revisit your G-Spot Symptom checker. Set new baseline numbers and keep these handy for when you get to your goal.

Want more? This might be the perfect time to take us up on our offer for more support. In the Resources and References section below you can learn more about how we can take you to the next level. Remember, we are here for you and want to be a part of your success!

If you have lost the weight, then the first order of business is…

Yahoo! Savour this moment! It must feel good and you should be incredibly proud.

Our suggestions for success going forward:

1. **Choose a buffer.** Realistically, you will not maintain the EXACT same weight day in and day out. What you can do is choose a buffer zone around your current weight.

   For example, if you are now at 130 lb., your buffer zone could be anywhere from 125 to 135 lb. Maybe you buffer zone is only 2 or 3 lb. above and below your current weight. No matter the number, make sure that you are comfortable with this. Check in weekly on the scale. If your weight is outside of your buffer zone, then that is your signal to rein things in a bit. Perhaps you need to start tracking your foods again? Skip the treats for a week or get back into a regular routine at the gym. You set the buffer and self-regulate.

2. Be flexible. Now that you have made it, you have a bit more flexibility in terms of your food choices. Here's what I mean: as long as you are following the plan 80 percent of the time or more, you should be able to maintain your weight. Keep in mind the first few weeks of maintenance will be a little rocky, so check in often and you will find your groove.

3. Fill out your G-Spot Symptoms Checker you can download this and other resources here: http://bonus.weightlossgspot.com/ . Also fill out your weight and measurements (refer to Chapter 3 for a reminder on how to do this). Please take an "after" picture of yourself and compare the two sets of pictures and how much you have changed so far.

4. Now write your "Before" and "After" measurement numbers in the table below and compare the two sets of numbers. Look at the differences in your weight, your measurements, even how many fewer symptoms you checked off the second time around on the symptom checker. My guess is that many nagging complaints have lessened or gone away completely.

	WEIGHT	WAIST MEASUREMENTS	HIP MEASUREMENTS
BEFORE			
AFTER			

*To attain a very lean, thin look, if you haven't already, get into the gym. This will help tone and tighten and get you to that next level.

5. Spread your wings. The world is your oyster. You have conquered something so few people do and we hope this gives you the courage and motivation to keep setting new personal goals for yourself.

Whether athletic, spiritual, professional etc., keep making yourself your best YOU. The clean eating lifestyle program outlined in this book will keep your body fueled for anything that comes your way.

In these next steps, we see you living your life more fully, feeling better than you have ever before, guiding and coaching loved ones with the lessons you have already mastered, having more self-love and self-awareness, self-acceptance, self-care, peace and much more. Remember! YOU need to take care of you—and that's why there is so much reference to "self" in our acknowledgement of what mastery looks like.

Your next journey starts now!

Isn't that so exciting? I hope you think so, too.

With all our hearts, we wish for you nothing but health and happiness and we are so thrilled to have been a part of this transformation with you.

Your "G" team,

Michelle and Nancy xo

RESOURCES

Shopping List for Pillar 1

Here is a list of all potential groceries you will need:

- Eggs

- Stonemill or Ezekiel (Food for Life) bread

- Protein powder (see list from Chapter 5)

- Unsweetened rice/coconut/almond/soy/hemp milk (optional)

- Berries, fresh or frozen

- Ground flax seeds

- Baby spinach

- Cottage cheese 0% or plain Greek yogurt 0%

- Nuts or seeds (any): options include sunflower, pumpkin or sesame seeds, slivered almonds, pistachios

- Cinnamon

- Plain quick oats

- Tuna (2-3 tins)

- Extra virgin olive oil

- Greens lettuce leaf

- Fresh lemon

- Avocado

- Mustard

- Mustard

- Chicken breast

- Bell peppers

- Chickpeas (canned or soaked)

- Onions

- Red wine vinegar

- Dried spices like oregano and basil

- Olives

- Goat feta cheese

- Pita (whole wheat or gluten free)

- Hummus (bought or homemade)

- Raw veggies (your choice)

Recipes from Chapter 7:

Granola

- 2 ½ cups rolled oats

- ¼ cup sunflower seeds

- ¼ shredded unsweetened coconut

- ¼ cup pumpkin seeds

- 1 tbsp. cinnamon (feel free to add more)

- ¼ tsp. sea salt

- 2 tbsp. coconut oil

- ⅓ cup raw honey or agave

- **Add 3 tbsp. Hemp hearts over each individual serving

Preheat the oven to 300F.

In a large bowl mix all dry ingredients.

In a small bowl combine honey and coconut oil, pour over dry mix and combine well.

Spread mixture over parchment-lined baking sheet and bake for 20 min, flipping around after 10 minutes.

Continue baking until your preference or the mixture is a golden brown.

Store in airtight containers like a mason jar.

Paleo Pancake

- 1 large banana, very ripe with black spots on skin

- 1 whole egg and 2 egg whites

- ½ tsp. cinnamon

- ¼ tsp. nutmeg

- 1 tbsp. hemp seeds

- ⅛ tsp. baking soda

- *optional: 1 tablespoon almond butter (or peanut butter, if you prefer)

Preheat your oven to 400F and line a baking sheet with parchment paper.

In a small bowl, mash the banana until it resembles a puree, then mix in the egg, baking soda, cinnamon, nutmeg, nut butter and hemp until well incorporated.

Using a spoon, drop the batter onto the lined baking sheet into 4 evenly sized pancakes. (I used about 2 spoonfuls per pancake)

Bake for 12-15 minutes at 400F, or until golden brown.

Serve warm with fresh fruitTropical Twist Smoothie

- ¼ ripe fresh mango, peeled and diced

- ¼ cup diced fresh pineapple

- 6 frozen strawberries

- 1 ½ cups (375mL) water or rice milk or other milk substitute

- 1 serving protein powder

- 1 tbsp. (15mL) flaxseed oil or hempseed oil or coconut oil

Put all the ingredients in a food processor or blender and pulse until smooth, adding more liquid if necessary.

Almond Joy, Raspberry Bliss Smoothie

1 cup frozen mixed berries (strawberries, blueberries, and raspberries)

½ cup (375mL) almond milk (unsweetened)

1 tablespoon (15mL) almond butter

½ tsp. almond extract

1 serving protein powder (see options from Chapter 5)

1 cup water

Icc (optional)

Combine ingredients into a blender and enjoy!

Raspberry Almond Smoothie

- 1 cup Raspberries

- ½ cup almond milk (unsweetened)

- 1 Tbsp almond butter

- Pinch of cinnamon

- ½ tsp almond extract

- 1 serving protein powder

- 1 cup water

Savoury Sage and White Bean Dip

- 3 tbsp. olive oil

- 1 large garlic clove, minced

- 1 can white kidney beans, drained and rinsed

- ¼ cup finely diced sun dried tomatoes, in oil, drained

- ¼ cup toasted pine nuts or pecans

- 1 tbsp. fresh chopped sage leaves

- Sea salt and pepper to taste

Blend together- white kidney beans, 3 tbsp. olive oil and garlic until smooth in a food processor or with an Emerson blender.

Stir in sage, sun dried tomatoes and toasted pine nuts to mixture until well combined.

Serve with Mary's crackers, Ryvita crackers or with veggies!

Power Smoothie

- 1 ½ cups water (or more)

- ¼ cup freshly juiced fruit (organic apple juice) *optional

- Handful of spinach

- 1-2 tsp. coconut oil/extra virgin olive oil

- ½ cup fresh or frozen berries

- 1-2 tsp. of chia (salba seed)* optional

- 1 serving of a good quality protein powder

Blend together and enjoy!

Turkey/Chicken Chili

- 1 lbs minced turkey or1 lbs skinless chicken breast, cubed

- 1 sweet onion (chopped)

- 3 tbsp. grape seed or olive oil

- 1 can lentils (rinsed)

- 1 can black beans (rinsed)

- 1 20oz canned or fresh diced tomatoes

- Pinch cayenne pepper

- 1 tsp. cumin

- 1tsp. garlic powder

- ½ tsp. dried oregano

- 1 tsp. sea salt

- ½ tsp. ground pepper

Sautee onions and meat until browned (this gives them more flavour).

Transfer all of the ingredients to slow cooker or large stove-top pot.

Stir in remaining ingredients.

Cover and cook over low heat for 3-5 hours.

Enjoy!

Makes 4 servings

Beet Salad

- 4 beets (greens removed but skin left)

- ½ tsp. cinnamon

- 1 ½ tsp. sugar

- 2 tbsp. lemon juice

- 2 tbsp. extra virgin olive oil

- salt

- 2 tbsp. chopped parsley

Preheat oven to 425F. Line a baking sheet with foil.

Place beets on prepared baking sheet and roast until fork tender, about 1 hour.

Let beets cool. Peel beets and roughly chop.

While beets are cooling, whisk together cinnamon, sugar, lemon juice, and olive oil in a large bowl. Add beets and stir to combine. Season with salt to taste.

Let beets rest in refrigerator for at least one hour. When ready to eat, take beets out of refrigerator and let come to room temperature. Sprinkle beets with parsley and serve.

Recipe from: Yummly.com

Vegetable Power Protein Soup

- 1 chicken (organic preferably) or vegetable stock pack

- 4 diced celery stalks

- 2 diced sweet onions

- 2-3 diced carrots

- 1tsp. garlic powder

- 2-3 garlic cloves

- 1 tbsp. olive oil

- ½ cup of brown rice or quinoa (uncooked)

- 1 can of lentils or chickpeas (rinsed)

- A cup of fresh or frozen peas

- ½ cup chopped parsley

- Sea salt and pepper to taste

Sauté the carrots, celery, garlic and onions with olive oil in a soup pot over medium-high heat.

Cover until they soften, about 5 minutes. Add the broth, rice (or quinoa) and lentils (or chickpeas) and garlic powder.

Bring the works to a simmer and continue cooking until the rice and lentils are tender, about 30 minutes.

Just before serving, stir in the peas and parsley. Cook just long enough to heat them through.

Serving: 4-6 Servings

Fruit Mint Salad

- 2 apples, cored and cubed

- 1 cup blueberries or blackberries

- 1 fresh mango, peeled and cubed OR 1 cup chopped strawberries

- 1 lime, juiced

- 1 tbsp. Pure natural liquid honey - I like the brand: Dutchman's Gold

- 6 fresh mint leaves, thinly sliced into ribbons

- ¼ cup unsweetened coconut

In a large bowl, combine apples, mangos and berries.

Mix together lime juice and honey. Microwave on high for 15 to 20 seconds to soften honey. Pour mixture over fruit. Add mint and gently toss to combine.

In a dry skillet, toss coconut over medium heat until lightly toasted, 5 to 7 minutes. Sprinkle over fruit salad right before serving

Serves 4

Recipe inspired from: Inspired Magazine

Onion and Spinach Salad

Slice two sweet or Spanish onions thinly. Place in a sauté pan. Turn the heat to low medium and allow onions to slowly brown and caramelize. Once cooked to your liking add desire amount to a bed of fresh spinach and top with shrimp.

Drizzle with 1 tsp. olive oil and sprinkle with sea salt for your dressing

Spaghetti Squash

Cut in half length-wise and remove seeds.

Place on a cookie sheet in the oven, on 400F, facedown.

Once squash becomes fork tender (about 45 min) remove from oven.

With a fork, shred the squash until you get long strings of squash that can be used instead of pasta noodles

Sweet Potato Fritata

- 1 large sweet potato cut into thin round slices

- 8 eggs whisked

- 1 tsp. garlic powder

- 2-3 garlic cloves

- 1 tbsp. olive oil

- ½ cup of brown rice or quinoa (uncooked)

- 1 can of lentils or chickpeas (rinsed)

- A cup of fresh or frozen peas

- ½ cup chopped parsley

- Sea salt and pepper to taste

Sauté the carrots, celery, garlic and onions with olive oil in a soup pot over medium-high heat.

Cover until they soften, about 5 minutes. Add the broth, rice (or quinoa) and lentils (or chickpeas) and garlic powder.

Bring the works to a simmer and continue cooking until the rice and lentils are tender, about 30 minutes.

Just before serving, stir in the peas and parsley. Cook just long enough to heat them through.

Serving: 4-6 Servings

Island Alive Smoothie

- 6-7 ice cubes

- 1/2 cup unsweetened almond milk (or coconut milk)

- 3 tbsp hemp seeds

- 1/2 tsp vanilla extract

- 3/4 cup fresh pineapple

- 1 tbsp almond butter

- 1/2 tsp maca powder (optional)

- 1/2 fresh lime squeezed

- * add more water or ice for a thinner consistency

Blend and enjoy!

Do You Need A Push? We Are Here To Help!

Option #1 Food-Based Accountability

If you are someone who needs that extra little bit of support and accountability in the food department, this is for you!

What you get:

Individualized support from me, Michelle, your nutritionist!

Weekly accountability to help you achieve Your Weight Loss G-Spot

A personalized review of food logs, plus comments for improvements

Peace of mind, knowing that you're making awesome decisions!

Want to know more? Contact Michelle at michelle@strongnutritionandweightloss.com

Option #2 Own It In My Soul Accountability

If you've been nodding your head in recognition and agreement throughout this book so far, but haven't started your journey yet, it's time for some coaching that will kick start your head and your heart into action!

What you get:

Six individual coaching sessions from me, Nancy, your Connection Coach

Daily accountability check-ins (as needed)

This book's content, customized to your individual needs through coaching

The support of someone who gets it, with the ability to help you overcome self-created hurdles

Want to know more? Contact Nancy at Nancy@nancymilton.ca

DISCLAIMER

None of the information contained in this book, whether it is our opinion, the opinion of the experts in this book or the additional resources made available constitutes, or substitutes for, medical advice.

If you are pregnant, diabetic, or have any life-threatening health challenges, please talk to a qualified health care professional first before undergoing any program described in this book.

We disclaim all responsibility, loss, or risk, personal or otherwise, that is incurred as a consequence, directly or indirectly, of the use and application of any of the content of this book or any additional resources that have been made available.

REFERENCES

Dr. Seuss. (1990) Oh, The Places You'll Go. 1990. Random House. 1

Schawbel, D. (2013, December 17).Dan. 14 Things Every Successful Person Has In Common. Forbes Retrieved from, 17 December 2013.http://www.forbes.com/sites/danschawbel/2013/12/17/14-things-every-successful-person-has-in-common/

Canfield. J. (2005).Jack. The Success Principles: How to Get from Where You Are to Where You Want to Be. 20052005William Morrow Paperbacks2005, p. 251.

Despres, J.P,Jean-Pierre Després, PhD. (2012). , FAHA, FIAS. Body Fat Distribution and Risk of Cardiovascular Disease: An Update...;. 2012; 126: 1301-1313 doi: 10.1161/CIRCULATIONAHA.111.067264

Your Journey to Better Health: A Step-by-Step Guide. FirstLine Therapy Lifestyle Medicine Programs by Metagenics. ppPgp. 18, 2013.

Turner, N. (2011). The Hormone Diet. Random House Canada. ppP381p. 381.

Boyles, S. WebMD (2004). Drinking Water May Speed Weight Loss. WebMD. Retrieved from http://www.webmd.com/diet/news/20040105/drinking-water-may-speed-weight-loss

Trigger."n.d" In Dictionary.com online. Retrieved from Dictionary.Com dictionary.reference.com/browse/trigger

A.M Davis, 1736.

Mittleman, S. (2001).Stu. Slow Burn.2000 Avon2000. p. 216-217.

Tabas,I.,& Glass, C.K. (2013, January 11). Anti-Inflammatory Therapy in Chronic Disease: Challenges and Opportunities. , Ira Tabas, Christopher K, Glass, Science ,11 January 2013: Vol. 339 no. 6116 pp. 166-172

DOI. 10.1126/science.1230720

Davis, W. Wheat Belly: Lose The Wheat, Lose The Weight and Find Your Path Back to Health. (2011). Collins.

Montried,P. Weizman, A. Kook, K. Morrow, A,L. Paul, S. (1993 May). Repeated swim-stress reduces GABAA receptor α subunit mRNAs in the mouse hippocampus. Molecular Brain Research. Volume 18, Issue 3, P 267–272. Retrieved from http://www.sciencedirect.com/science/article/pii/0169328X9390199Y

The Mayo Clinic. (2013) Chronic Stress Puts Your Health At Risk. Retrieved from http://www.mayoclinic.org/healthy-living/stress-management/in-depth/stress/art-20046037

Turner, N. (2011). The Hormone Diet. p.Random House Canada. P94p. 94.

Jon Kabat-Zinn (1990). Zindel, Segal, et al, 2012.

Stener-Victorin,E. & Wu,X. (2010, October 28). Effects and mechanisms of acupuncture in the reproductive system. The Journal of Autonomic Neuroscience: Basic and Clinical. Vol 157(1):46-51,doi:10.1016/j.autneu.2010.03.006.

Elisabet Stener-Victorin a,b,!, Xiaoke Wu b.

Louise Hay, L. (1999). You Can Heal Your Life,,. Hay House., 1999, p. 9.

Joy. "n.d" In Merriam- online Webster dictionary online. Retrieved from www.merriam-webster.com/dictionary/joy. online

Trimarchi, M. Why are New Year's resolutions so easy to break? Retrieved from http://people.howstuffworks.com/culture-traditions/holidays-other/new-year-resolutions-easy-to-break.htm

33621124R00193

Made in the USA
Middletown, DE
20 July 2016